5

88 participants. 1 [illegible]

W. Martin — TB in USA & Canada

(Go to end of world to learn

in own backyard!!)

— El Paso [illegible] — all >1000 [illegible]

[illegible] daily operations.

[illegible] of [illegible] cattle [illegible] adjoining [illegible]

Next: ~~28–30~~ 29–31 March '95 READING

SOCIETY FOR VETERINARY EPIDEMIOLOGY AND PREVENTIVE MEDICINE

Proceedings of a meeting held at the Queen's University of Belfast on the 13th, 14th and 15th of April 1994

Edited by M.V. Thrusfield

ISBN 0 948073 14 4

ACKNOWLEDGEMENTS

Secretarial assistance in collating the proceedings was provided by Mrs R. Hunter and Mrs R. Muirhead.

The following companies provided financial support for the conference and for publication of these proceedings:

Cyanamid UK

Dickinson & Co

Genus Animal Health

Lilly Indiustries Ltd

MSD Agvet

Norbrook Laboratories (GB) Ltd

Northern Ireland Tourist Board

Pedigree Petfoods

Rhone Merieux

Roche Products Ltd

Ross Breeders

SmithKline Beecham Animal Health Limited

Solvay Duphar Veterinary

Univet

Veterinary Business Development

Webster Animal Health

CONTENTS

TUBERCULOSIS

THE DIAGNOSIS OF BOVINE TUBERCULOSIS BY BLOOD TESTING

S.D. Neill*, J. Hanna*, J. Pollock*, D.P. Mackie*, J. Cassidy*, A. Clements** and D.B. Bryson*

Bovine tuberculosis can still be significantly damaging to local and in some instances national farming economies throughout the world. The various diagnostic tests available and associated field data from several countries have been recently reviewed by Monaghan (in press) and O'Reilly (in press). Most eradication programmes rely on intradermal tuberculin testing, as it is generally assumed that this will ensure that virtually all tuberculous cattle are detected early in the infection. Whilst these tests are considered effective in many countries, some national programmes of tuberculosis eradication have encountered difficulties in removing the final residue of bovine infection. In these countries potential reservoirs for the infection have usually been sought amongst local wildlife.

Although much of the research on bovine tuberculosis was discontinued following successful eradication programmes in several developed countries, research interest has recently been renewed. Immunological responses to *M.bovis* infections in cattle are being studied in an attempt to develop improved or alternative diagnostic methods, as skin testing has practical drawbacks and is not without controversy in relation to sensitivity and specificity.

Currently there is no universally accepted diagnostic blood test for tuberculosis in cattle. The ELISAs for antibody detection (Hanna et al., 1989, 1992; Plackett et al., 1989) may have limited diagnostic value considering the significance of the cell mediated response in tuberculous cattle (Thorns and Morris, 1983; Neill et al., 1991). *In vitro* determinations of cell mediated responses have generally relied on the lymphocyte proliferation assay, however a simple ELISA for bovine interferon-gamma has now been developed as an alternative (Wood et al., 1990; Rothel et al., 1991).

As a spectrum of immune responses can follow *M.bovis* infection (Neill et al. 1991), there is possibly diagnostic potential both for assays able to detect humoral and cell mediated responses in blood. This paper reports the findings from a preliminary study in which the potential of several laboratory assays to diagnose bovine tuberculosis was being assessed. The results from the blood assays are compared with those from traditional skin testing.

---

*The Veterinary Sciences Division, Department of Agriculture (N. Ireland), Stormont, Stoney Road, Belfast BT4 3SD, Northern Ireland.

**The Veterinary Services Division, Department of Agriculture (N. Ireland), Dundonald House, Belfast BT4 3SB, Northern Ireland.

MATERIALS AND METHODS

This study was a preliminary evaluation and was carried out with certain constraints. To obtain the maximum number of diseased cattle from the minimum number of animals tested, the study targeted cattle which gave inconclusive reactions in their last skin test and those considered "at risk" from contiguous contact with known infected herds or from contact with infected animals moved into the herd. Herds which were historically free from tuberculosis for at least the previous five years were also included.

Skin test

Cattle were skin tested in the field using the single intradermal comparative cervical test in accordance with recognised procedures (EC directive 80/219/EEC amending Directive 64/432/EEC, Annex B). Bovine and avian PPD antigens (Central Veterinary Laboratory, Weybridge) were used throughout the study. All of the animals were examined clinically at the time of skin testing. Only those animals which had not been skin tested during the previous sixty days were included in the study.

Blood assays

Cattle were always bled prior to skin testing. Blood (8-10ml) was collected into vacutainers containing lithium heparin (143 u.s.p. units) and submitted to the laboratory for examination within 6 hours bleeding. Bloods were processed and assayed by ELISAs for antimycobacterial antibodies and interferon-gamma, and for lymphocyte proliferation as described previously (Neill et al., 1992).

Skin test reactors were taken for compulsory slaughter at a designated abattoir. Where possible, cattle which gave a positive response in a blood assay but were unresponsive in the skin test were purchased for extensive post-mortem and laboratory examinations.
Specimens of heparinised blood and nasal mucus (usually 1-2ml) were taken from animals immediately before slaughter and submitted for laboratory examination.

Post-mortem examinations

Thorough meat inspection procedures were carried out on all abattoir slaughtered animals and the retropharyngeal, bronchial, mediastinal and mesenteric lymph nodes were dissected out. These, together with any suspect lesions, were submitted to the laboratory for histopathological and bacteriological examinations.

Detailed post-mortem examinations were performed on the cattle which were skin test negative but positive in a blood test. Lesions suspect of skin tuberculosis were taken for histopathological examination. Retropharyngeal, submaxillary, parotid, bronchial, mediastinal, mesenteric and supramammary lymph nodes were dissected free and sectioned at 2mm intervals. Samples from all of these nodes and any suspect lesions found were taken for histopathological and bacteriological examinations. Both lungs were carefully examined externally, lavaged and specimens submitted for laboratory examinations. The head was divided longitudinally along its midline and a careful inspection made of the nasal mucosa, turbinates, nasal septum, nasopharynx, pharyngeal and palatine tonsils. Samples of all these tissues were taken for histopathological and bacteriological examinations.

Histopathological examinations

These were carried out as described previously (McIlroy et al., 1986).

Bacteriological examinations

Bacteriological examinations were carried out as previously described (Neill et al., 1988). All specimens were processed and cultured individually. Lung washings and specimens from the anterior respiratory tract were also cultured biologically using guinea pigs.

Animals were considered diseased when *M.bovis* was isolated and/or histopathological examinations confirmed tuberculosis. When no tuberculous lesions were found at post mortem and *M.bovis* was not isolated from specimens, the animals were considered not to be diseased.

RESULTS

During the study, 4195 cattle were tested. Of these, 2799 cattle were targeted as potentially diseased and 1007 cattle were from herds apparently free of tuberculosis. Three hundred and eighty nine non tuberculous cattle at a local abattoir were also tested.

One hundred and fifty-three cattle from the target group were recorded as reacting positively in the tuberculin skin test. Only 74 of these cattle were identified using standard interpretation of the test. Table 1 shows the proportions of skin reactors which were scored positive in each of the blood assays.

There were 89 diseased or infected cattle detected during the study and Table 2 shows the numbers of these which were identified by the individual tests. Typical tuberculous lesions were observed grossly in lymph nodes associated with the respiratory tracts. Lesions were confirmed tuberculous by histopathological examination and isolation of *M.bovis*.

All of the cattle from the "tuberculosis-free" herds and those selected at the abattoir were skin test negative. Cattle, from the target group and the tuberculosis free herds, which showed no responses in both the skin tests and blood assays were not slaughtered. No evidence of tuberculosis was observed at routine meat inspection of the cattle selected at abattoir slaughter. Table 3 shows the estimated specificities for each of the tests employed in the negative populations.

There are obviously many permutations which can be considered when comparing the skin test and blood test results. As the ELISA for interferon-gamma produced the highest number of blood positive results for the skin test negative animals, most effort was therefore directed towards obtaining those skin test negative cattle which had an interferon response. Of the animals targeted as potentially diseased, 196 were positive in the interferon assay and of these 98 had no skin reaction. It proved difficult to obtain the skin test negative cattle which were blood test positive, as compulsory purchase was not possible. Of the 98 interferon positive/skin test negative cattle detected, only thirty-nine animals were made available for post-mortem examinations.

Fourteen (35.9%) of these 39 animals had tuberculous lesions and/or *M.bovis* cultured from specimens. One animal from the TB-free herds was also positive in the interferon assay and was purchased. Post-mortem revealed tuberculous lesions and *M.bovis* was isolated. Table 4 shows a summary of the significant laboratory findings for these 15 skin test negative cattle. The lesions were small (approx., 1-2 mm in diameter), and usually no more than one lesion site in each animal was found. Of the initial fourteen animals, twelve had been recorded as "inconclusive" at their previous skin test (a mean test interval of 66 days) and a further two were from restricted herds (test intervals of 61 and 63 days). The fifteenth animal (number 3348) was identified during an annual herd test (test interval of 388 days) of cattle with a record of being free from tuberculosis for at least 5 years.

DISCUSSION

The constraints on carrying out this preliminary evaluation were such that the true sensitivities and specificities of the tests were unattainable. Many of the animals in the blood test positive category and most cattle in the "negative" population were not subjected to post-mortem examinations. Additionally, whilst the extensive post-mortem and laboratory examinations of some blood test positive cattle yielded extremely valuable information, the procedures for examining the cattle selected from the skin test and blood test results were obviously not uniform. Despite these drawbacks, the estimated specificities for the tests (Table 2) show several tests as being acceptable for field application. The blood assays identified the majority of the cattle which were positive in the skin test. The skin test detected a number of diseased animals not identified by the blood tests. However there was a greater number of diseased cattle detected by the interferon ELISA which failed to respond when skin tested. The calculated sensitivities for the interferon ELISA and the skin test (severe interpretation) were similar (84.3% and 83.1% respectively). Although this finding was extremely encouraging, the numbers of diseased cattle detected during the study was unfortunately insufficient to allow an adequate degree of confidence in the comparison of the tests. The results confirm that applying the standard interpretation to the interdermal tuberculin test used in a high risk population will fail to detect all diseased animals (sensitivity was 55.1%).

Respiratory lymph node tissues represented a significant proportion of the specimens in which lesions were found or from which *M. bovis* was isolated. The detection of small usually single tuberculous lesions in seven of the 15 animals from which *M. bovis* was isolated and the absence of lesions in the remaining eight cases would indicate early infection. The isolation of *M. bovis* from tissues such as tonsil, nasal pharynx, trachea, and nasal mucus (Table 4) serves to emphasise the potential of these animals to shed the organism and transmit infection. More than one third of the group of the 39 skin test negative animals examined were shown to harbour *M. bovis* in respiratory secretions and lymph nodes.

It is known that some cattle with generalised tuberculosis fail to respond to skin testing. Fortunately, the number of such "anergic" cattle in a population which has been subjected to regular skin testing over many years is generally low. The present study has now demonstrated a significant number of cattle in the early stages of infection, which also fail to respond to skin testing. It is not known when or if these cattle would become reactive to the intradermal tuberculin test, but their existence has significant implications for epidemiological studies on bovine tuberculosis

Table 1a. Number of skin test positive cattle detected by each test

Skin test (Standard)	IFN assay	T3 assay	T5 assay	Eppd	Ephos
153 (100%)	94 (61.4%)	70 (45.8%)	50 (32.7%)	10 (6.5%)	45 (29.4%)

Table 1b. Number of skin test positive cattle detected by each test

Skin test (Standard)	IFN assay	T3 assay	T5 assay	Eppd	Ephos
74 (100%)	61 (82.4%)	45 (60.8%)	34 (45.9%)	7 (9.4%)	17 (22.9%)

Skin Test:	Single comparative intradermal tuberculin test.
Standard Interpretation:	$\geq$5 mm bovine bias; severe interpretation: includes $\geq$3 mm bovine bias.
IFN assay:	ELISA for bovine interferon-gamma.
T3/T5 assays:	Lymphocyte transformation assays carried out over 3 and 5 days respectively.
Eppd/Ephos:	ELISAs incorporating PPD and Phosphatide antigens respectively for detecting humoral antibodies.

Table 2. Number of diseased cattle detected by each test

Skin test (severe)	Skin test (standard)	IFN assay	T3 assay	T5 assay	Eppd	Ephos
74 (83.1%)	49 (55.1%)	75 (84.3%)	51 (57.8%)	40 (45%)	4 (4.8%)	24 (27%)

Table 3. "Specificity" of each test

Skin test	-	100%
IFN assay	-	99.6%
T3 assay	-	94.1%
T5 assay	-	87.3%
Eppd	-	97.5%
Ephos	-	88.5%

Table 4. Post-mortem and histopathological findings from culture positive skin test negative cattle

Animal number	Post-mortem[a]	Histopathology[a]	Culture
9	-	-	+(l)
541	b,m	b,m	+(b,m,p)
690	-	-	+(m)
692	-	-	+(b,r,m)
1579	-	-	+(nm)
1589	-	-	+(p)
1721	r	r	+(r)
2006	m	m	+(m)
2263	-	-	+(np,nm,tr)
2266	-	-	+(m)
3348	b,m	b,m	+(b,m)
3897	-	-	+(m)
4245	m	m	+(m)
4272	b	b	+(b,m,t)

[a]Tuberculous lesions observed in the specimens shown.
+ M.bovis isolated from specimens shown.

Specimens:-

b = bronchial lymph node; m = mediastinal node; r = retropharyngeal nodes; p = parotid; np = nasal pharangax; t = tonsil; tr = trachea; nm = nasal mucus and l = lung lavage and its ultimate eradication from the national herds. Despite the obvious benefit of detecting early tuberculosis, general employment of the interferon-gamma assay must await evaluations of its sensitivity and specificity from a significantly larger number of cattle. Such a study is currently being completed in N. Ireland.

REFERENCES

Hanna, J., Neill, S.D., and O'Brien. (1989). Research in Veterinary Science. 47, 43.

Hanna, J., Neill, S.D., and O'Brien. (1992). Veterinary Microbiology. 31, 243.

McIlroy, S.G. Neill, S.D. and McCracken, R.M. (1986). Veterinary Record. 118, 718.

Monaghan, M.L.M. (In press). Pathogenesis of Mycobacterium bovis in cattle. Veterinary Microbiology.

Neill, S.D., O'Brien, J.J. & McCracken, R.M. (1988). Veterinary Record. 122, 184.

Neill, S.D., O'Brien, J.J. & Hanna, J. (1991). Veterinary Microbiology. 28, 103.

Neill, S.D., Hanna, J., Mackie, D.P. and Bryson, T.G.D. (1992). Veterinary Record. 131, 45.

O'Reilly, L.M. (In press). Pathogenesis of Mycobacterium bovis in cattle. Veterinary Microbiology.

Plackett, P., Ripper, J., Corner, L.A., Small, K., de Witte, K., Melville, L., Hides, S. and Wood, P.R. (1989). An ELISA for the detection of anergic tuberculosis cattle. Australian Veterinary Journal. 66, 15-19.

Rothel, J.S., Jones, S.L. Corner, L.A., Cox, J.C. and Wood, P.R. (1990) Australian Veterinary Journal. 67, 134.

Thorns, C.J. and Morris, J.A. (1983). The immune spectrum of *Mycobacterium bovis* infections in some mammalian species: A review. Veterinary Bulletin. 53, 543-550.

Wood, P.R., Corner, L.A., Rothel, J.S., Baldock, C., Jones, S.L., Cousins, D.B., McCormick, B.S., Francis, B.R., Creeper, J. and Tweddle, N.E. (1991). Australian Veterinary Journal. 69 (9) : 286.

BOVINE TUBERCULOSIS AND THE CONTRIBUTION OF A TUBERCULOUS BADGER POPULATION

L.A. DOLAN[1] J.A. EVES[2] AND D.H. WILLIAMS[3]

A national Bovine Tuberculosis Eradication (BTE) scheme commenced in the Republic of Ireland in 1954. The programme was based on a test and slaughter policy using the single intradermal comparative tuberculin test (SICTT) as the principal method of diagnosis. In 1965 the country was declared attested when the test failure rate had fallen from an initial estimated figure of 17 per cent of animals to 0.5 per cent (Watchorn, 1965). In the intervening years limited progress has been made towards the goal of eradication (Downey, 1990). During this time the cattle population increased from an estimated 4.3 million in 1950 to an estimated 6.9 million in 1980 (Central Statistics Office, 1986) and has remained close to this figure to date.

In the early 1980's field investigations of outbreaks of bovine tuberculosis suggested that tuberculous badgers were involved on a number of farms. Badger removal was subsequently undertaken on a trial basis in selected areas. These trials involved herds in five counties located in the midlands, west and south of the country. There was a definite and substantial decrease in both herd breakdown rate and test reactor animals identified, subsequent to these badger removals. However, comparable control areas, in which badgers had not been removed, had not been monitored in the same period (O'Connor and O'Malley, 1989).

Post-mortem examination of 3,909 badgers carried out in the Republic of Ireland, between 1980 and 1989, disclosed a gross lesion rate of 17 per cent (Dolan and Lynch, 1992). Most of the badgers were captured, under licences issued by the Wildlife Service, in areas that had experienced extensive outbreaks of tuberculosis in the associated cattle populations. Consequently, the disease level recorded in the badgers may not have been representative as it was recorded in a selected sample of badgers. The remaining badgers were either road casualties or were found dead on farms. Tuberculous badgers were identified in every county in the country during that period.

A National Badger Survey, commenced in 1989, has recently been completed. The preliminary results indicated that the adult badger population in the Republic of Ireland was approximately 200,000 (Smal, 1993).

In their review entitled "Badgers and Bovine Tuberculosis in the Republic of Ireland", O'Connor and O'Malley (1989) concluded that eradication of bovine tuberculosis might not be achieved in parts of the country unless the associated tuberculous badger population was controlled. Likewise Morris and Pfeiffer (1990), in a consultancy report prepared for the Eradication of Animal Disease Board (ERAD), concluded that the tuberculous badger population was causing special difficulties in the bovine tuberculosis eradication programme.

[1] Tuberculosis Investigation Unit, University College, Dublin 4.
[2] Dept. Agriculture, Food and Forestry, Tullamore, Co. Offaly.
[3] Department of Statistics, University College, Dublin 4.

A large scale observational study of the effects of badger removal on the rate of disclosure of tuberculosis in herds in a designated area in the midlands commenced in 1989. The study is entitled the East Offaly Badger Research Project (EOP). This paper describes the progress of the project to-date.

MATERIALS AND METHODS

Study area

The area selected for the study was primarily in the eastern part of Co. Offaly but extended into parts of three adjoining counties (Figure 1). The area was comprised of some 738 sq. kms. as calculated by geographical information systems technology (GIS) (Hammond, R.F., personal communication). The boundary of the area, which was agreed between ERAD and the Wildlife Service, was outlined by rivers. In order to take account of badger immigration at the periphery of the study area, those farms situated within 1.5 kms. of the boundary were designated as being within a Buffer Zone. The remaining central area was then referred to as the Project Area and was comprised of 540 sq. kms.

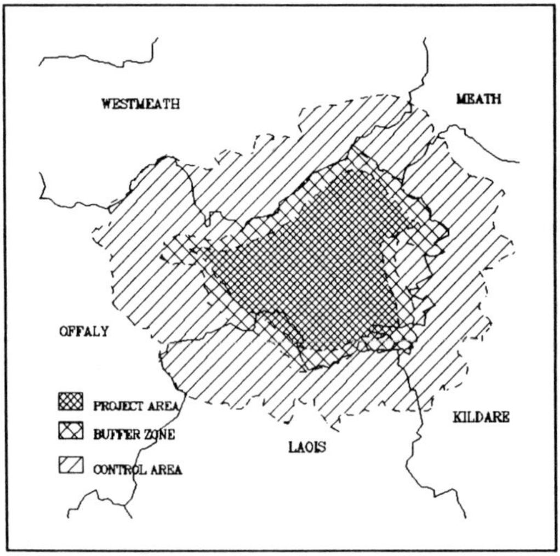

Figure 1. The Project Area, Buffer Zone and Control Area of the East Offaly Badger Research Project.

The areas immediately surrounding the badger removal area, to a depth equivalent to two District Electoral Divisions (DED's), were designated as a Control Area. The farms in this area provided, as far as possible, comparable cattle stocking rates and enterprise types. The size of a DED, in this rural area, was dependant on the human population which was, in turn, very dependant on farm size. The DED was primarily used for administrative purposes such as the issuing of herd numbers, area testing, etc.

Badgers

The badger removal area was surveyed prior to the study to identify setts and badger activity. The approved method of capture of the badgers was by snaring; they were then euthanised by shooting with a small bore rifle. The snaring was carried out systematically, area by area. Once snares were placed they were revisited at twenty four-hour intervals until removed. Following capture the badgers were tagged, sexed, weighed and then delivered to a Regional Veterinary Laboratory where they were subjected to post-mortem examination (Eves, 1994).

Cattle

There were approximately 1,000 active herds, containing approximately 55,000 cattle, in the Project Area each year. The figures for the Control Area were approximately 2,900 herds and 145,000 animals, respectively. These data were generated from the national computer recording systems at the various county District Veterinary Offices (DVO's). Herd details for the Buffer Zone were excluded from the analysis.

Tuberculin testing data

For the purposes of the study the tuberculin testing results, at both herd and animal levels, for the Project and Control Areas were compared. Tuberculin testing data were available for all herds in both areas from 1982. Initial results were recorded against 1988 as the reference year. The overall testing regime was comparable in both areas each year. Herds in which reactors were disclosed were retested at 60-day intervals until two successive clear tests were achieved. Each herd was then listed for a six-month check test.

Analysis

In order to remove the effect of herd size the herds were divided into quartiles, for the purposes of more detailed analysis. Herd sizes in each group were 1-17, 18-39, 40-76 and >76 animals. Data for this analysis were available from 1982 for both areas. The herd breakdown rate was calculated for each area in each year.

For each year and for each group of herds (and all herds) the number of herds in the Project and Control Areas having a breakdown, i.e., with one or more reactors to the tuberculin test, was recorded, and a two-way table comparing the two areas was analysed using a chi squared test.

For herds having a breakdown, the maximum number of reactors identified at a single test in a year was used as the variable to compare herds within each group (and all herds) between the Project and Control Areas, using a t-test.

A number of statistical models were considered to assess factors that might affect the incidence of herd breakdown, including herd size and the existence of a previous breakdown. Other factors in the two areas were considered to be equal in effect. With herd size included in the model, a previous breakdown was found not to be significant and so the latter factor was not included in the final model, which related the chance of a breakdown to a function of herd size in a logistic regression analysis. The logistic model was found adequate for describing the chance of a breakdown in herds of less than 77 cattle.

RESULTS

A total of 1,508 badgers were captured in the four years, 1989 to 1992. Twelve per cent of these showed evidence of tuberculosis on gross post-mortem examination (Table 1). Over half the total number of badgers were caught in the first year. The number of badgers captured in the third and fourth years represented 23 and 22%, respectively, of the number captured in 1989.

Sixteen percent of the badgers were caught in the Buffer Zone in 1989; in 1991 and 1992 this figure had risen to 39 and 40%, respectively. It would appear from these figures that, using the present method of capture, it may not be possible to reduce the number of badgers inhabiting the Buffer Zone and the Project Area, primarily due to immigration. The percentage of tuberculous badgers had decreased from 14 per cent in 1989 to 5 per cent by 1992.

Table 1. The number of badgers trapped and the number found to be tuberculous in the Project Area and Buffer Zone. East Offaly Project, 1989 to 1992 inclusive.

Year	Project Area	Buffer Zone	Total
1989	700	137	837
	*94 (13)	25 (18)	119 (14)
1990	197	103	300
	24 (12)	3 (3)	27 (9)
1991	117	74	191
	13 (11)	8 (11)	21 (11)
1992	108	72	180
	7 (6)	2 (3)	9 (5)
Total	1122	386	1508
	138 (12)	38 (10)	176 (12)

* number and percentage ( ) of badgers found to be tuberculous on gross post-mortem examination.

There was a 68 per cent reduction in the total number of reactors identified within the Project Area in 1992 compared to the 1988 figure (Table 2). There was a decrease of 21% in the Control Area in the same period, though there had been an increase each year initially to a maximum of 34% in 1991. The reactor disclosure rate per 1,000 animal tests carried out in 1992 in the Project Area, at 1.37, represented a fall of 63 per cent compared to the 1988 rate, while that observed in the Control Area in 1992, at 2.45, represented a fall of 15 per cent in the same period.

Table 2. The number of tuberculin reactors, APT and per cent change, by year, in the Project and Control Areas of the EOP, from 1988 to 1992.

Year	Area	No. of Reactors/year		APT/year*	
1988		321		3.72	
1989	Project	343		3.34	
1990		281		2.87	
1991		176		2.54	
1992		102	(-68)	1.37	(-63)
1988		720		2.89	
1989	Control	829		3.09	
1990		789		3.18	
1991		966		4.51	
1992		567	(-21)	2.45	(-15)

* Reactor animals per 1,000 animal tests
( ) % change from 1988 figure.

From 1982 to 1990, herd breakdown rates were higher, though not significantly so, in the Project Area than in the Control Area. In both 1991 and 1992, however, this rate was significantly lower in the Project Area (Table 3). When subgroups of herds were analysed the same overall pattern was observed, with significantly lower breakdown rates for herds with <18 animals in 1991 and with 18-39 animals in 1992.

Analysis of the mean number of reactors disclosed per breakdown showed that in 1982 the mean number of reactors was significantly greater in the Control Area ($P<0.05$) and was marginally higher in 1983. From 1984 to 1989 this figure was greater for the Project Area, but not significantly so. In the years 1990, 1991 and 1992 the mean number of reactors was less in the Project Area, and significantly so (Table 4) for the latter two years ($P<0.05$).

Table 3. The breakdown probability for herds in each year and each herd size grouping for the Project and Control Areas.

		Breakdown Probability				
		Herd Size				
		<18	18-<40	40-<77	>77	All
Year	Region					
88	Project	0.051	0.067	0.177	0.191	0.111
	Control	0.045	0.091	0.148	0.192	0.110
89	Project	0.047	0.114	0.115	0.245	0.124
	Control	0.037	0.095	0.134	0.243	0.119
90	Project	0.047	0.065	0.173	0.188	0.112
	Control	0.057	0.071	0.132	0.197	0.110
91	Project	**0.018**	0.075	0.087	0.223	**0.099**
	Control	**0.074**	0.103	0.122	0.230	**0.131**
92	Project	0.028	**0.022**	0.082	0.098	**0.055**
	Control	0.032	**0.066**	0.081	0.143	**0.079**

Boldface values differ significantly (P < 0.05)

In 1991 and 1992 the risk curves based on the logistic analysis (i.e., plots of the chance of a breakdown against herd size) were found to differ significantly between the two areas (P<0.01). The only significant difference observed prior to 1991 was in 1987, when herds in the Project Area had a greater breakdown rate (P<0.05). For 1991 the curves ran in parallel, increasing by herd size to approximately 50 animals. The curves then came together at approximately 70 animals. In 1992 the curves were together at a herd size of 5 animals, then separated out with the curve for the Project Area increasing very gradually until a herd size of 50 animals, when the curve rose quickly to meet the descending Control Area curve at a herd size of 60 animals.

A preliminary inspection of data for the first six months of 1993 indicates a continuation of the downward trend in both herd breakdown and reactor numbers for both the Project and Control Areas.

Table 4. The mean number of reactors identified, at a single tuberculin test, in each year and each herd size grouping for the Project and Control Areas, 1988 - 1992.

Mean number of Reactors

Herd Size

Year	Region	<18	18-39	40-76	>76	All
1988	Project	1.24	2.76	2.03	3. 0	2.37
	Control	1.45	1.86	2.04	3. 0	2.30
1989	Project	1.75	1.76	3.33	2.79	2.52
	Control	1.51	1.66	2.35	2.58	2.24
1990	Project	2.06	1.93	1.82	2.65	2.19
	Control	1.76	1.92	2.38	2.97	2.45
1991	Project	1.50	1.81	**1.38**	2.54	**2.12**
	Control	1.89	2.55	**2.39**	3.68	**2.89**
1992	Project	**1.00**	1.40	1.53	2.36	**1.77**
	Control	**1.40**	2.20	2.40	2.70	**2.37**

Boldface values differ significantly ($P < 0.05$)

DISCUSSION

The badger removal programme undertaken in the East Offaly Badger Research Project provided an effective means of controlling the resident badger population, for the purpose of the project. The programme, however, was not effective in preventing the immigration of badgers into the area. No appreciable reduction in the rate of disclosure of tuberculosis in captured badgers occurred over the period (Table 1), and the continuing occurrence of the disease in badgers captured in both the Project Area and the Buffer Zone must be taken into account when analysing the results.

There was a decrease in both the herd breakdown rate and the mean number of reactor animals per breakdown, in the Project Area as compared to the Control Area, both in 1991 and 1992, i.e. years 3 and 4 of the study. Likewise a lower rate of disclosure of reactors to the tuberculin test was seen in the Project Area, as compared to the Control Area, for the same period. These findings indicated that the extent of tuberculosis in the herds in the Project Area had declined relative to that in the Control Area, in the latter part of the study.

As the supervised removal of badgers is the one differentiating feature between these two areas, it is reasonable to consider the possibility that badger removal and an improvement in the tuberculosis status of herds in the area were related. Such a conclusion has been advanced in other studies reviewed by O'Connor and O'Malley (1989). The East Offaly Project which was undertaken as an observational study, will provide further data for consideration.

The patterns of distribution of the badger here, as reported by Smal (1993), indicated that the extent of contact with cattle may be greater than in Great Britain. The occurrence of *Mycobacterium bovis* strains having the same REA characteristics in badgers and cattle, in six of the nine outbreaks investigated provided further evidence of the extent of contact between these two animal species (Collins *et al.*, 1993). In the present study, there also appears to be an association between the likelihood of a breakdown and the proximity of a herd to a badger sett in areas in which tuberculous badgers have recently been captured (Dolan *et al.*, 1994). Contiguity with other herds which are concurrently undergoing an outbreak has been described as characteristic of some breakdowns in Ireland (O'Connor *et al.*, 1993); however, it is not clear if this is the result of cattle-to-cattle transmission of *M. bovis*, or the result of exposure to a single point source, such as infected wildlife.

The East Offaly Badger Research Project, when completed, is expected to provide useful information on the effectiveness of badger removal as a means of protecting herds from infection from tuberculous badger populations.

ACKNOWLEDGEMENTS

The authors wish to thank the staff at the District Veterinary Office, Co. Offaly for their continuing contribution to the project; the staff of the Tuberculosis Investigation Unit, University College Dublin for their assistance and criticisms and Mr. Cormac McLean, Statistics Department, University College Dublin for his contribution to data assembly and analysis.

REFERENCES

Central Statistics Office (1986). Statistical Abstract, 1982-85, P. 81. Stationery Office, Dublin.

Collins, J.D., Collins, D.M., DeLisle, G.W. and Costello, E. (1993). Typing of *Mycobacterium bovis* Isolates from Cattle and Badgers in the Same Locality. Selected Papers, 1992, pp 37-38. Tuberculosis Investigation Unit, University College, Dublin.

Dolan, L.A. and Lynch, K. (1992). Badgers and Bovine Tuberculosis. Selected Papers, 1990 - 1991, Tuberculosis Investigation Unit, University College Dublin.

Dolan, L.A., Hammond, R.F., Eves, J.A., Griffin, J.G., Collins, J.D. and Martin, S.W. (1994). The Association between Distance to Badger Setts and Badgers, and Bovine Tuberculosis Reactor Status of Herds in East County Offaly, 1988 - 1992. In Selected Papers, 1993. Tuberculosis Investigation Unit, University College Dublin. In press.

Downey. L. (1990). In " Ireland's TB problem - What Can and Must Be Achieved". Eradication of Animal Disease Board, Dublin.

Eves, J.A. (1994). Proceedings of the Royal Irish Academy Symposium on the Badger, Dublin, April 1991. In press.

Morris, R.M. and Pfeiffer, D. (1990). Consultancy Report on the Bovine Tuberculosis Eradication of Animal Disease Board, Dublin.

O'Connor, R. and O'Malley, E. (1989). In " Badgers and Bovine Tuberculosis in Ireland". Economics and Social Research Institute, Dublin.

O'Connor, R., Conway, A. and Murphy, M. (1993). In "Study of Socio Economic Impediments to Bovine Tuberculosis Eradication". Economic and Social Research Institute, Dublin.

Smal, C. (1993). In " The Badger and Habitat Survey of Ireland". The Wildlife Service Office of Public Works, Dublin.

Watchorn, R.C. (1965). In " Bovine Tuberculosis Eradication Scheme (1954 - 1965)". Stationery Office, Dublin.

OPEN SESSION

THE EPIDEMIOLOGIST'S AND PRACTITIONER'S ROLE IN FOOD QUALITY ASSURANCE SYSTEMS

Th. Blaha*

Modern quality assurance systems not only check the quality of the final product, they also assure 'production of quality' at every stage in the production chain. In the case of pork production, up to now, most attention has been focussed on slaughter; the breeding, rearing and finishing periods have not been involved in quality assurance.

In this paper, an epidemiological information system is presented. It indicates herd health status and provides a basis for purposeful veterinary consultation with the farmer.

The first step in extending quality assurance to herd level is identification of an indicator of herd health. One quite sensitive indicator is the quantity of gross pathological lesions in the lung, pleura, pericardium and liver.

Table 1 shows the system for recording the kind and severity of possible lesions to be found in individual slaughtered pigs.

Table 1. Evaluation of lung lesions in individual animals

Lesions	*Symbol*	*Definition/ decision taken*
Pneumonias:		
- light	Pn 1	< 10%
- medium	Pn 2	11 - 30%
- severe	Pn 3	> 30%
Pleuritis:		
- light	Pl 1	> coin-size
- medium	Pl 2	coin-size to palm-size
- severe	Pl 3	> palm-size
Pericarditis	Pc	Present
Milkspots:		
- light	L 1	trimming
- severe	L 2	condemnation

*Department of Epidemiology, Veterinary School of Hanover, Buescheler Strasse 9, D-49456 Bakum, Germany.

Table 2 demonstrates evaluation of the health status of slaughter-pig groups, calculating the percentage of lung lesions, pleuritis and pericarditis per slaughter-pig group. For example, if a group of 100 pigs included one pig with medium pneumonia (coded Pn 2 in Table 1) and two pigs with severe pneumonia (coded Pn 3) then 3% of pigs in the group would have either medium or severe pneumonia, and the group would be awarded two 'points' in Table 3. The use of points allows aggregation of different pulmonary lesions to produce a summary indicator of 'batch' health: herds with 0 points having the best 'respiratory health', and herds with 16 points having the worst.

Table 2. Key for using lung lesions as indicators of herd health

Percentage of pigs/group with medium and severe pneumonia (Pn 2 + Pn 3)	*Points*	*Percentage of pigs/group with medium and severe pleuritis (Pl 2 + Pl 3)*	*Points*	*Percentage of pigs/group with pericarditis (Pc)*	*Points*
<1	0	<1	0	<1	0
1 - 20	2	1 - 10	1	1 - 5	1
21 - 40	4	11 - 30	2	6 - 10	2
41 - 70	6	31 - 50	3	11 - 15	3
>70	8	>50	4	>15	4

Thus, classes for the health status of herds can be defined:

0-3	points	= very good
4-6	points	= good
7-9	points	= moderate
10-13	points	= poor
14-16	points	= very poor.

The continuous recording of these data on the frequency and severity of lesions in slaughter pigs of the herds delivered to one slaughter house produces a rough survey of the health status of these pig herds. Table 3 shows two examples of such a survey.

The average results of the slaughter-pig groups from one herd over longer periods (e.g., six months) will inform the farmer of the long-term health status of his herd, and he will be able to compare this status with that of the herds of other farmers (Table 4).

Pig owners that repeatedly 'earn' points higher than 9 will look for pieces of advice, since they know of, or are informed about, the reduction of the pigs' performance by diseases causing lesions that still can be found at slaughter. If the veterinary practioner is prepared to support the farmer in improving his herd health management,

Table 3. Health assessment of batches of slaughter pigs from two herds

Batch health	*Milkspots*	*Limb injuries*	*Stuffed stomachs*	*Beating marks*
Herd 1:				
11 points	L1 = 10%			
= poor	L2 = 0%	17%	34%	0%
Herd 2:				
2 points	L1 = 22%			
= very good	L2 = 34%	0%	0%	37%

Table 4. Herd health in the period from... to...

Herd health					
Own herd	*All herds in the region**				
11 points = poor	0-3 very good	4-6 good	7-9 medium	10-12 poor	13-16 very poor
	8%	53%	29%	6%	4%

*Percentages refer to the proportion of herds in each point category.

animal hygiene, housing conditions, early recognition of diseases and monitoring herd health status, he will be a permanent partner in modern production chains for pork. The epidemiological comparison of herds with high health status with those of low health status will increase the epidemiologists' and practitioners' ability to improve and maintain the health of pig herds.

INTER-RELATIONSHIPS OF PERIPARTURIENT DISEASES IN DAIRY COWS

E.J. PEELER, M.J. OTTE, and R.J. ESSLEMONT[1]

Events around the time of calving are crucial in determining future reproductive success. Many of these events inevitably occur as a 'complex' (Curtis et al., 1985). The relationships between periparturient diseases in dairy cattle have been assessed using data from North America (Erb et al., 1985; Dohoo & Martin, 1984) and Sweden (Oltenacu et al., 1990).

Erb et al. (1985) and Curtis et al. (1985) found that dystocia increased the risk of vulval discharge (VLD), but not retained foetal membranes (RFM). However, Gröhn et al. (1990) reported that cows which were assisted at calving were four times more likely to retain their fetal membranes than cows which were not assisted. Most authors (Erb et al. ,1985; Gröhn et al. ,1990; Curtis et al., 1985) have remarked on the greatly increased risk of VLD in cows with RFM. Gröhn et al. (1990) also reported that dystocia, acute mastitis and lameness were significant predictors for VLD, whereas Markusfeld (1984) found that twinning and stillbirth were important risk factors for the condition. Anoestrus, cystic ovaries and inactive ovaries have been associated with high milk production (Bartlett et al. ,1987), twinning (Markusfeld ,1987; Emanuelson & Bendixen, 1991) and VLD (Erb et al., 1985; Pepper & Dobson, 1987).

Diseases occurring around the time of calving are important on economic and welfare grounds. This paper describes the relationships between periparturient conditions derived from data from 10 British dairy herds.

MATERIALS AND METHODS

Data from 3603 lactations were obtained over three seasons (1988/89 - 1990/91) from 10 autumn calving, commercial dairy herds in the south west of England, all of them using the same veterinary practice and computerised recording system (DAISY, The Dairy Management and Information System, University of Reading).

The herds consisted of Friesian-Holstein stock and the average herd size was 120 cows, ranging from 69 to 230, with an annual milk yield of 5500 to 6300 kg/cow. The data were examined to ensure that the standard of disease recording was consistent and complete.

[1] Veterinary Epidemiology and Economics Research Unit, Department of Agriculture, University of Reading, Earley Gate, Reading RG6 2AT.

A case of VLD was defined as a discharge consisting of at least 50 per cent purulent matter. RFM was defined as retention for at least 24 hours after calving and calf mortality was defined as any calf born dead or dying within 24 hours of birth. Cows receiving assistance at calving by the farmer or the veterinary surgeon were recorded as cases of dystocia. Lameness and mastitis were diagnosed by the farmer.

Any cow examined by the veterinary surgeon because of a failure to observe her in oestrus was classified as a case of oestrus not observed.

Statistical Analysis

In the simplest form, an odds ratio is the ratio of odds of a disease occurring in individuals exposed to a particular determinant and the odds of the disease occurring in individuals not exposed to the determinant. An odds ratio of one implies no association, a ratio significantly greater than one indicates a positive association and a ratio significantly less than one indicates a negative association with the determinant. Simple comparisons may lead to biased estimates of odds ratios if two or more conditions, which are themselves associated, constitute determinants of a disease. As a result, multivariate statistical techniques are required to assess the possible role of a given determinant, while controlling for the effects of the other determinants present. The conditional odds ratios, calculated from the partial regression coefficients derived from logistic regression, are adjusted for all the other factors included in the regression model.

A logistic regression analysis was performed with each disease condition as the dependent variable, using the 'Statistix' program (version 4; Analytical Software). Diseases were represented as binary variables. A disease was only introduced as a predictor variable if the relationship tested appeared chronologically sensible; i.e. twinning could plausibly lead to dystocia but dystocia could not be a causative factor for twinning. Some relationships could be two-way; for example dead calves could be a putative factor for dystocia and vice versa, whereas other relationships may be mere associations, eg, mastitis before service and lameness before service. 'Parity' and 'herd' were represented by dummy variables in all regressions. The factor 'parity' was coded in such a way that parities 2, 3, 4 and greater than 4 were compared with parity 1; the factor 'herd' was coded so that odds for a particular herd were compared with the overall 'average' odds for all the herds. Regression models with interactions between parity and the predictor variables, and between predictor variables themselves were examined. The statistical significance of the decrease in deviance for the model with an interaction was assessed by a X^2 test.

RESULTS

The overall lactational incidence rates for different diseases and traits, together with the rates in each parity are given in Table 1. The incidence rates for each parity are controlled for herd. Table 2 shows the lactational incidence rates for each herd, and Table 3 shows the conditional odds ratios for the predictor variables that were significant at the 5 per cent level.

Odds ratios are also given for first calvers and multiparous cows where the decrease in deviance, in the model with parity interactions, was significant at the 5 per cent level.

Table 1. Variations with parity in the incidence rates of diseases and traits among 3603 lactations in 10 herds during three calving seasons

	Lactational incidence rates (%)[a]					
Disease or trait	Total (3603)	Parity 1 (742)	Parity 2 (572)	Parity 3 (552)	Parity 4 (519)	Parity >4 (1218)
Vaginal discharge	25.3	33.4	19.6	23.1	22.8	23.5
Retained fetal membranes	4.4	3.0	2.6	2.5	4.2	5.3
Dystocia	12.9	18.1	8.6	9.3	11.3	8.7
Calf mortality	6.1	8.4	4.9	3.9	3.4	4.1
Twinning	3.3	0.7	2.3	5.1	5.0	4.1
Pre-service lameness	8.9	4.4	6.1	4.9	8.3	13.6
Pre-service mastitis	14.4	6.5	10.8	10.9	14.0	21.9
Oestrus not observed	37.1	41.7	36.3	40.6	36.7	32.7

[a] Incidence rates for each parity are controlled for herd.

Twinning and calf mortality were investigated as predictor variables for dystocia, but only calf mortality was significant (odds ratio 2.10). Twinning and dystocia were significant predictor variables for the death of one or both calves (odds ratio 2.92 and 2.02, respectively).

Twinning was the only factor which significantly increased the risk of RFM (odds ratio 5.92). Twinning, dystocia, calf mortality, and most importantly RFM all increased the likelihood of VLD (odds ratios 5.41, 1.77, 2.55 and 11.70).

Twinning, dystocia, RFM, and lameness before service all had significant odds ratios for mastitis before service (odds ratios 1.61, 1.39, 1.92 and 1.44 respectively). Dystocia and mastitis before service were significant predictors for lameness before service (odds ratios 1.47 for both predictors).

The most important predictor for oestrus not observed was twinning (odds ratio 1.59). VLD and lameness diagnosed before service were also significant predictors (odds ratios 1.28 and 1.42 respectively), lameness being particularly important in first calvers (odds ratio 3.66). The only significant negative association observed was between calf mortality and oestrus not observed (odds ratio 0.59).

Table 2. Variations in the incidence rate of diseases and traits among 10 herds over three calving seasons and 3603 lactations.

Disease or trait	Lactational incidence rates (%)[a]									
	Herd 1	Herd 2	Herd 3	Herd 4	Herd 5	Herd 6	Herd 7	Herd 8	Herd 9	Herd 10
Vaginal discharge	28.0	17.7	26.7	15.4	21.8	26.2	19.9	35.7	25.9	36.3
Retained fetal membranes	1.0	3.0	6.3	2.7	2.1	2.2	25.0	5.3	4.2	3.5
Dystocia	9.6	11.9	14.1	8.9	4.0	14.3	32.1	2.0	16.1	36.0
Calf mortality	5.0	4.3	4.1	2.3	4.6	10.7	7.7	8.8	1.4	10.5
Twinning	4.6	3.4	2.1	4.6	3.1	5.0	4.5	2.5	5.6	3.3
Pre-service lameness	21.1	14.1	6.8	7.4	7.7	6.0	2.6	5.5	18.9	7.0
Pre-service mastitis	34.5	22.7	27.4	19.3	22.9	34.9	35.9	17.3	21.0	37.6
Oestrus not observed	38.5	29.9	50.1	32.4	26.8	38.5	32.1	47.5	50.3	36.1

[a] Incidence rates for each herd are controlled for parity.

Table 3. Conditional odds ratios for the inter-relationships of variables

Predictor	Outcome						
	Dystocia	Calf mortality	Retained fetal membranes	Vaginal discharge	Pre-service mastitis	Pre-service lameness	Oestrus not observed
Twinning		2.92	5.92	5.41	1.61		
Dystocia	*	2.02		1.77	1.39	1.47	
Calf mortality	2.10	*		2.55			0.59
Retained fetal membranes	*	*	*	11.90	1.92		
Vaginal discharge	*	*	*	*			1.28
Pre-service mastitis	*	*	*	*	*	1.47	
Pre-service lameness	*	*	*	*	1.44	*	3.66[a] 1.42 1.19[b]

* Relationships not tested
The odds ratios are all significant at the 5% level, except that marked by [b] which also indicates an odds ratio for multiparous cows.
[a] indicates an odds ratio for primiparous cows.

DISCUSSION

The highest incidence rates of dystocia, calf mortality, oestrus not observed and vulval discharge occurred in first calvers (Table 1). Thompson et al. (1983) also found that calf mortality and dystocia occurred most commonly in first parity cows; they also reported that there was no association between age at first calving and dystocia, but they recorded more severe dystocia in smaller first parity cows.

The highest incidence rates for mastitis (22.0 %) and lameness before service (13.6 %) were observed in cows with parities greater than 4 (Table 1). The incidence rate of RFM was lowest in parities two and three, 2.56 % and 2.54 %, respectively.

Erb et al. (1985) argued that heifers should be considered separately because their diseases and reproductive parameters are different from those of multiparous cows. In this study the only significant interaction detected was between parity and lameness diagnosed before service. However, many of the conditions occurred at low incidences, which reduces the power to detect significant relationships, and the problem is exacerbated by the reduced size of the samples when separate parities are considered.

Dystocia showed the largest between herd variation of any of the variables, the incidence ranging from 2.0 % to 36.0 % (Table 2). This wide range can partly be explained by variation in the willingness of the herdsman to assist, as well as by vriations in the necessity to do so, and by the variation in criteria used by herdsmen to define a case.

The influence of management policy and husbandry is reflected by the variation between herds in the incidence of lameness (2.6 % to 21.1 %), mastitis (17.3 % to 37.0 %), calf mortality (1.45 % to 10.7%), and VLD (15.4 % to 35.7 %). Nine of the herds had an incidence rate of less than 6% for RFM, but the other herd had an unusually high rate, 25 %. Twinning had a predictably small variation in incidence between herds, from 2.1 % to 5.6 %.

Twinning has been associated with high milk yield (Wood, 1984). The relationships between high milk production and mastitis (Bartlett et al., 1987; Bunch et al., 1984) and oestrus not observed (Emanuelson & Bendixen, 1991; Markusfeld, 1987; Bartlett et al., 1987) may partly explain why twinning was associated with increased odds ratios both these conditions (odds ratios 1.61 and 1.59 respectively). The results of this study are in agreement with Markusfeld (1987) who reported that twinning was the most important factor leading to inactive ovaries. It is possible that the relatively poorer body condition at calving which is associated with twinning, could lead to an increased susceptibility to mastitis and poor fertility. The greatly increased risk of RFM in cows that had twins (odds ratio 5.92) could have been due to a shorter gestation length (the gestation length was not recorded in this study) and uterine inertia.

The increased risks of calf mortality, RFM and VLD after delivery of twins (odds ratios 2.92, 5.92 and 5.41) were in agreement with Markusfeld (1987). Eddy et al. (1991) attributed the increased incidence of a VLD after twinning primarily to the increased incidence of RFM.

In common with Erb et al. (1985) and Curtis et al. (1985) dystocia was found to be a significant predictor for VLD (odds ratio 1.77). Gröhn et al. (1990) found that dystocia carried a risk of RFM but not VLD. This study did not find that dystocia was associated with significant risk of RFM. Erb et al. (1985) only found that dystocia was associated with a risk of RFM only in primiparous cows (odds ratio 4).

Dystocia was a significant risk factor for mastitis and lameness diagnosed before service (odds ratios 1.39 and 1.47). It is possible that a traumatic delivery could have a debilitating influence and thus have increased the cow's susceptibility to disease. Milian-Suazo et al. (1989) found that dystocia was a significant predictor for culling due to foot or leg lameness. They speculated that a poor conformation of the pelvis could predispose cows to both conditions or that assistance at calving had lead to obturator or tibial nerve damage, and thus lameness.

There was also an association between dystocia and calf mortality (odds ratios 2.02 and 2.10). Thompson and Rege (1984) found that 60 % of calves dying at birth had been delivered with assistance.

In this study calf mortality was a risk factor for VLD (odds ratio 2.55) in agreement with Markusfeld (1987), who, in contrast to this study, also found that calf mortality was a risk factor for RFM. The decomposition of a dead calf before delivery will inevitably result in the contamination of the uterus, and the trauma to the reproductive tract associated with the delivery of a dead calf, will predispose the uterus to the successful establishment of a uterine infection.

The negative association between calf mortality and oestrus not observed (odds ratio 0.59) may indicate that a cow, having delivered a dead calf, was allowed a longer period before being presented as not having been seen in oestrus.

RFM increased the likelihood of mastitis, but not lameness, before service (odds ratio 1.92). Curtis et al. (1985) have associated RFM with ketosis (odds ratio 16.4), but it is not clear which condition came first. It seems likely that some cases of RFM could also predispose the cow to mastitis.

There are clear biological reasons why RFM should be an important risk factor for a VLD. The odds ratio observed, 11.70, was higher than that reported by Erb et al. (1985), and Gröhn et al. (1989). However, Markusfeld (1984) considered that every case of RFM leads to a secondary VLD, and therefore speculated that some cases of primary VLD can be attributed to a 'hidden' RFM or to their retention for less than 24 hours.

A VLD was positively associated with oestrus not observed (odds ratio 1.28). Many studies have demonstrated a link between anoestrus and VLD (Halpern et al., 1985; Erb et al., 1985; Markusfeld, 1987). The measurement of milk progesterone concentration by Pepper and Dobson (1987) confirmed the link between chronic endometritis and a persistent corpeus luteum, but since high levels of the prostaglandin metabolite, 13,14-dihydro,15-ketoprostaglandin $F_{2\alpha}$, were also found, the life of the corpeus luteum was not prolonged by the lack of prostaglandin production. This implies the existence of another mediator or common factor(s) leading to both conditions.

Lameness and mastitis in the period before service were significantly associated (odds ratios 1.44 and 1.47). An environmental factor may predispose cows to both conditions, or a cow predisposed to one condition may have an increased susceptibility to the other. Alternatively, it is possible that having one condition predisposes a cow to the other.

Lameness before service increased the risk of oestrus not observed (odds ratio 1.42). Lameness could physically inhibit a cow from exhibiting oestrus behaviour, or if a lame cow were separated from the rest of the herd there would be less opportunity for it to express oestrus. The cow's ability to compete for food may be impaired by lameness, which could lead to anoestrus. Alternatively, high cortisol levels, resulting from pain-induced stress, might inhibit the release of luteinising hormone. The effect of lameness before service was greatest in first calvers (odds ratio 3.66). It is possible that first calvers suffer more severe lameness, or that cows in their first lactation are under a greater metabolic strain and are thus become anoestrus more easily. Oestrus not observed was recorded more frequently in first parity cows than in older cows (Table 1).

The major associations observed in this study were that twinning was the only significant predictor of RFM (odds ratio 5.92), and also a major predictor of VLD (odds ratio 5.41) and calf mortality (odds ratio 2.92). Calf mortality and RFM were the other two important predictors of VLD (odds ratio 2.55 and 11.70 respectively). Calf mortality and dystocia were strongly associated (odds ratio 2.0). There was good evidence to suggest that, when considering the inter-relationships of periparturient diseases, it would be worthwhile to consider separate models for different parities.

An assessment of the inter-relationships of periparturient diseases is necessary for the accurate evaluation of the economic costs of the diseases, as well as the formulation of an effective programme of preventive medicine. The large variations observed between herds for many of the conditions (Table 2) indicate that management and husbandry practices are important in determining the levels of disease. The cows' environment needs to be assessed in a consistent fashion in order to assess which influences are important.

Breed was found to be an important determinant of the associations between periparturient factors by Oltenacu et al. (1990) who found stronger links between dystocia, stillbirth, RFM and VLD for Swedish red and whites than for Swedish Friesians (odds ratios were about twice as large for the former breed). In addition to the relationships demonstrated in this study there is evidence that metabolic diseases should also be considered. Gröhn et al. (1988) have indicated that VLD and RFM could be direct risk factors for disorders of the abomasum and for ketosis. Markusfeld (1985) found a strong association between metritis and ketosis, and Curtis et al. (1985) found that the RFM, but not VLD, was an important risk factor for ketosis (odds ratio 16.4). Ideally investigations of inter-relationships between diseases should use data about the cows' nutrition and milk production that might indicate the underlying causes of disease.

ACKNOWLEDGEMENTS

We would like to thank the farmers and veterinary practice concerned for the data collection. Furthermore, we gratefully acknowledge the permission of The Veterinary Record to present the paper at this meeting.

REFERENCES

Bartlett P.C., Kirk J., Coe P., Marteniuk J. and Mather E.C. (1987). Descriptive epidemiology of anestrus in Michigan Holstein-Friesian cattle. Theriogenology 27, 459-476.

Bunch, K.J., Heneghan, D.J.S., Hibbit, K.G. and Rowlands, G.J. (1984). Genetic influences on clinical mastitis and its relationship with milk yield, season and stage of lactation. Livestock Production Science 11, 91-104.

Curtis R.C., Erb H.N., Sniffen C.J., Smith R.D. and Kronfeld D.S. (1985). Path analysis of dry period nutrition, postpartum metabolic and reproduction disorders, and mastitis in Holstein cows. Journal of Dairy Science 68, 2347-2360.

Dohoo I.R. and Martin S.W. (1984). Disease, production and culling in Holstein-Friesian cows V. Survivorship. Preventive Veterinary Medicine 2, 771-784.

Eddy R.G., Davies O. and David C. (1991). An economic assessment of twin births in British dairy herds. Veterinary Record 129, 526-529.

Emanuelson U. and Bendixen P.A. (1991). Occurrence of cystic ovaries in dairy cows in Sweden. Preventive Veterinary Medicine 10, 261-271.

Erb H.N., Smith R.D., Oltenacu P.A., Guard C.L., Hillman R.B., Powers P.A., Smith M.C. and White M.E. (1985). Path model of reproductive disorders and performance, milk fever, mastitis, milk yield and culling in Holstein cows. Journal of Dairy Science 68, 3337-3349.

Gröhn Y.T., Erb H.N., McCulloch C.E. and Saloniemi H.S. (1990). Epidemiology of reproductive disorders in dairy cattle: Associations among host characteristics, disease and production. Preventive Veterinary Medicine 8, 25-29.

Halpern, N.E., Erb H.N. and Smith R.D. (1985). Duration of retained fetal membranes and subsequent fertility in dairy cows. Theriogenology 23, 807-813.

Markusfeld O. (1984). Factors responsible for post parturient metritis in dairy cattle. Veterinary Record 114, 539-542.

Markusfeld O. (1985). Relationship between overfeeding, metritis and ketosis in high-yielding dairy cows. Veterinary Record 116, 489-491.

Markusfeld O. (1987). Inactive ovaries in high-yielding dairy cows before service: Aetiology and effect on conception. Veterinary Record 121, 149-153.

Milian-Suazo F., Erb H.N. and Smith R.D. (1989). Risk factors for reason-specific culling of dairy cows. Preventive Veterinary Medicine, 7, 19-29.

Oltenacu P.A., Frick A. and Linde B. (1990). Epidemiological study of several clinical diseases, reproductive performance and culling in primiparous Swedish cattle. Preventive Veterinary Medicine 9, 59-74.

Pepper, R.T. and Dobson H. (1987). Preliminary results of treatment and endocrinology of chronic endometritis in the dairy cow. Veterinary Record 120, 53-56.

Thompson J.R. and Rege J.E.O. (1984). Influences of dam on calving difficulty and early calf mortality. Journal of Dairy Science 67, 847-853.

Thompson, J.R., Pollack, E.J. and Pelissier, C.L. (1983). Interrelationships of parturition problems, production of subsequent lactation, reproduction, and age at first calving. Journal of Dairy Science 66, 1119-1127.

Wood, P.D.P. (1984). Some attributes of twin-bearing British Friesian and Canadian Holstein cows recorded in England and Wales. Journal of Dairy Research, 51, 365-370.

RELATIONSHIPS BETWEEN PIG HUSBANDRY PRACTICES AND VIOLATIVE DRUG RESIDUES

McCAUGHEY, W.J., McEVOY, J.D.G., CAMPBELL, J.N. KENNEDY, D.G. LYNAS, L.*
and
McCARTAN, B.M.**

Today the pig industry has a positive message to put across to health conscious consumers. Although still seen as a fatty food, carcases are leaner than ever before. Not only has the amount of backfat declined but the fat in lean has also reduced. In addition the fats in lean are more unsaturated. In this positive marketing situation it is vital that consumers should also be assured that the meat is produced with consideration for the welfare of the animals and with minimal, responsible drug use.

However there has been long standing concern over residues resulting from the use of antimicrobial drugs in pig production both as preventive therapies and as growth promoters. In Northern Ireland these concerns have been acknowledged and a regulatory programme to eliminate these from locally produced products began in 1986. The programme aims to provide quality assurance by regular testing of pigmeat and pigmeat products for residual concentrations of the commonly used veterinary antimicrobial drugs. Penalties are imposed as deterrents on producers who present pigs for slaughter containing concentrations of veterinary drug residues above the maximum residue limits (MRL).

MRL'S are set on the basis of an assessment of the safety of residues in feedstuffs for consumers continuously exposed to that level over a lifetime. The theoretical diets include higher than normal intakes of selected organs and incorporate a safety factor. These target concentrations provide a means of ensuring that acceptable daily intakes are not exceeded even by extreme consumers eating meat from properly treated animals. In Great Britain MRL's are specified in the Animals, Meat and Meat Products (Examination for Residues and Maximum Residue Limits) Regulations 1991 which came into force on 8 January 1992. It is expected that MRL's will eventually be established for most, if not all, veterinary drugs. In the Northern Ireland programme carcases which are shown to contain residues above the MRL are condemned.

The regulatory programme includes the collection of urine, kidney and muscle samples from one pig presented by each producer to the pig slaughter

* Veterinary Sciences Division, Stoney Road, Stormont, BELFAST, BT4 3SD, Northern Ireland.
** Veterinary Service, Dundonald House, Upper Newtownards Road, BELFAST. Northern Ireland.

plants in Northern Ireland on at least five occasions each year. The samples are stored at -20°C until analysed. The laboratory analyses include a screening sulphadimidine EIA test, a multi-sulphonamide HPTLC, a microbial inhibition test, high voltage electrophoresis bioautography, HPLC, LCMS and GC/MS. Positive results are used to target specific producers for more intensive sampling. In this second intensive stage a number of pigs, normally five, are sampled and the carcases are detained. The samples are examined by the same range of tests and carcases associated with those found to contain residues above the MRL are condemned. Producers remain on the intensive sampling schedules until they have achieved three completely clear tests. Condemnation of the carcases results in financial loss.

Implementation of this programme resulted in a sharp fall in the frequency of sulphadimidine residues above the MRL but has been less effective in reducing the frequency of positive antibiotic results. When violations occur the producer is visited by a veterinary officer from the Department of Agriculture to ascertain the probable reason for the violation and to provide advice on measures needed to avoid future loss. Information collected during these visits can be examined to determine changes in drug handling practices. This paper reports briefly on the progress of the scheme to detect antibiotic abuse and presents a summary of data from 1990-93 including 138 recent farm visit reports.

Data from animal feedingstuff antimicrobial analyses carried out in the laboratory over the same time interval have also been examined to indicate the level of antimicrobial cross-contamination which occurs during compounding. Experimentally this information has been used in experiments to investigate the importance of CTC in pig feeds.

ANTIMICROBIAL TESTS

There has been a small, non-significant, increase in the number of antimicrobial test positive samples identified in the random testing programme over the interval 1990 - 1993 (Table 1). These positives have involved both kidney and muscle tissues. The ratio between these two tissues is approximately 3:1 and has remained relatively constant.

Table 1. Microbial inhibition tests on randomly collected samples 1990 - 1993

Year	Total Tested	Total Positive	Kidney Positive	Muscle Positive
		%	%	%
1990	2959	136 (4.6)	136 (4.6)	33 (1.1)
1991	2870	110 (3.8)	110 (3.8)	40 (1.4)
1992	2533	115 (4.5)	115 (4.5)	33 (1.3)
1993	2510	126 (5.0)	126 (5.0)	44 (1.7)

From the start of the programme the antibiotic most frequently identified, following a microbial inhibition test positive result, was chlortetracycline (Figure 1). The details of all antibiotics identified

Figure 1. Results of Antibiotic tests on Pig Carcases

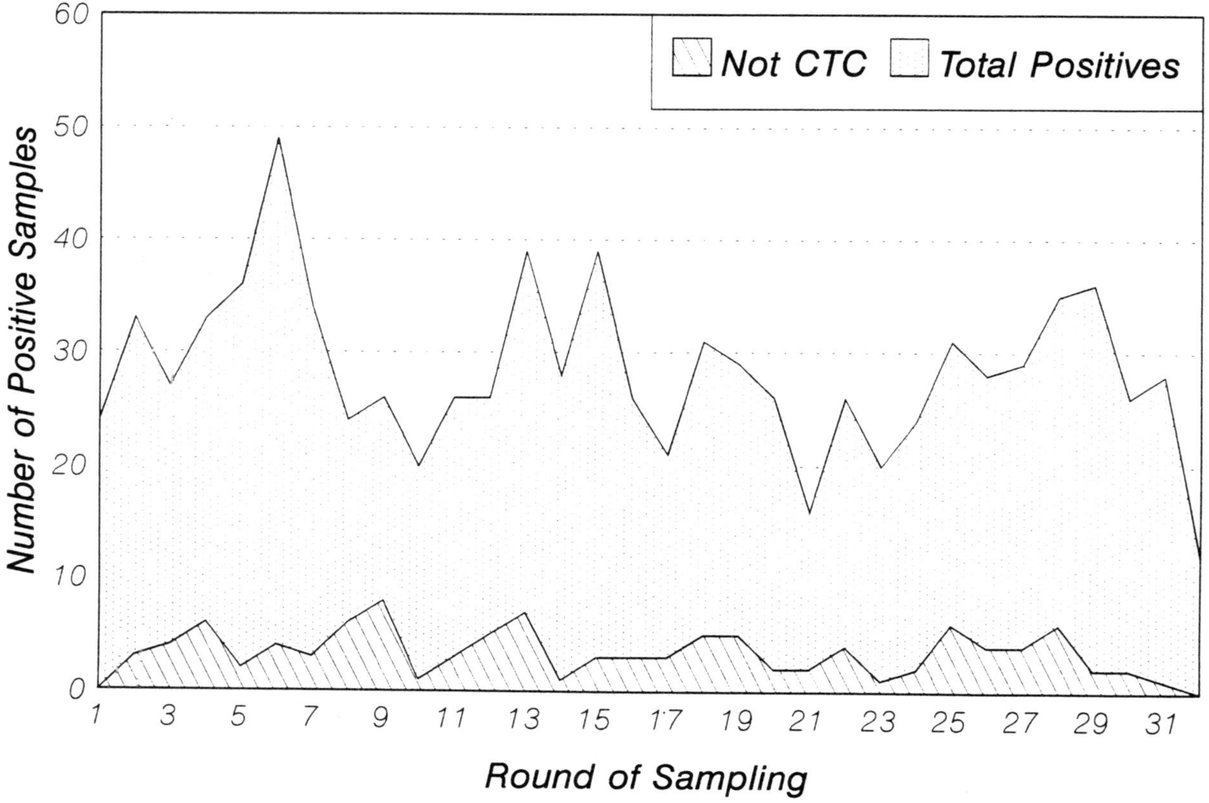

during 1990 - 1993 (Table 2) demonstrate that the pattern has been maintained.

Chlortetracycline is the most frequently reported antibiotic feed additive on pig farms and penicillin/streptamycin feature prominently in the field officers reports of drugs held on pig farms following the identification of positive carcases the random survey.

Table 2. Antibiotics identified following positive microbial inhibition tests on kidney samples. 1990 - 1993.

Antibiotic	Number of positive tests			
	1990	1991	1992	1993
Chlortetracycline	119	89	98	114
Streptomycin	10	12	13	8
Penicillin	3	2	.	1
Strepto/pen.	.	1	1	1
Oxytetracycline	.	1	.	.
Chlortet/pen	.	.	.	1
Lincomycin	.	.	3	.
Unidentified	4	3	.	.
TOTAL	136	108	115	125

The microbial inhibition test may identify antibiotic activity at concentrations which are below the current sensitivity of confirmation techniques. The low concentrations are responsible for the inability to identify all inhibitory substances. The number of samples in which the residue exceeded the MRL (Table 3) is considerably smaller than that in which the drug can be shown to be present (Table 2).

Table 3. Chlortetracycline residues exceeding the MRL 1990 -1993

Year	Total Tested	Kidney		Muscle	
		>0.6	%	>0.1	%
1990	2959	14	(0.47)	12	(0.40)
1991	2870	24	(0.83)	20	(0.69)
1992	2533	23	(0.90)	23	(0.90)
1993	2510	31	(1.23)	25	(0.99)

CHLORTETRACYCLINE

Chlortetracycline is consistently the most frequently identified antibiotic in pig tissue samples. The proportion of carcases found to contain residues of this antibiotic during the interval 1990 - 1993 and the ratio of positive results from paired kidney and muscle samples have remained relatively constant. The summarised results for 1993 (Table 4) show close agreement between the proportion of each tissue that exceed the MRL.

Table 4. Chlortetracycline concentrations in paired kidney and muscle samples (1993)

	Kidney	Muscle
MRL	0.6 ppm	0.1 ppm
Below the MRL	88	62
Above the MRL	31	25

The majority of confirmed positive chlortetracycline residues are below the MRL illustrating that the problems of chlortetracycline are more widespread than might be suggested by a study limited to those that are above the MRL. However the number of carcases condemned as a result of intensive testing and the number of producers penalised by these condemnations have remained low during the interval 1990 - 1993 (Table 5).

Table 5. Carcase condemnations resulting from violative Chlortetracycline residues

Year	Number of Carcases	Number of Producers
1990	23	8
1991	17	7
1992	23	6
1993	27	10.

FEEDINGSTUFFS TESTING

Samples of compounded animal feedingstuffs are collected from all registered compounders in Northern Ireland for analysis. During 1993 a total of 294 randomly collected animal feedingstuffs were tested. In 50 (17%) there were undeclared medications (Figure 2); of these 39 were identified as chlortetracycline the remainder were sulphadimidine (1), other sulphonamides (7), penicillin (1), avoparcin (1), tylosin (3) and in three cases the drug was not identified. The mean concentration and range in the chlortetracycline contaminated meals was 17.8 mg/kg (range <0.1 - 490 mg/kg). The range was discontinuous suggesting that contamination up to 30 mg/kg had occurred but that the 3 samples above this concentration may have been due to errors in compounding which had resulted in full therapeutic concentrations being added to the mix.

Figure 2. Contaminated Animal Feeding Stuffs 1993

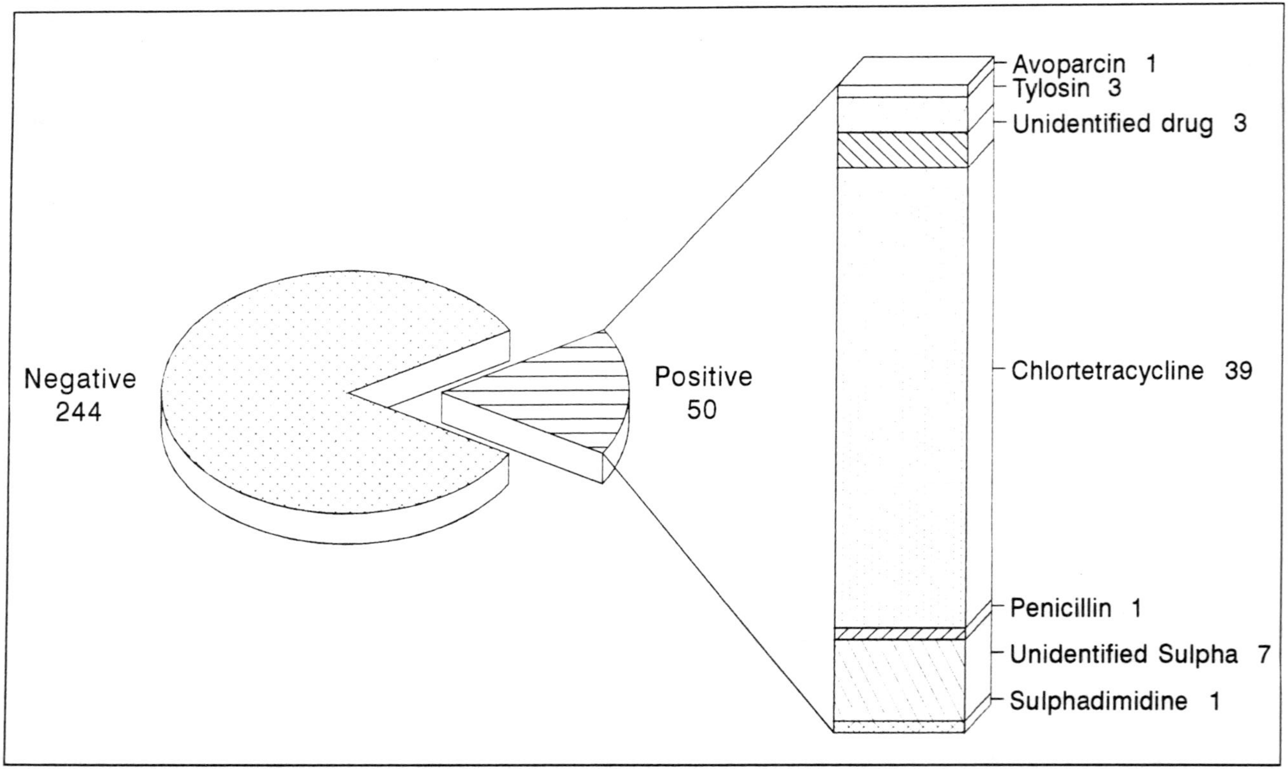

EXPERIMENTAL STUDIES ON CHLORTETRACYCLINE IN PIG PRODUCTION

As a result of the above observations 40 mg/kg was selected as a concentration suitable to study the effects of compounding contamination on the creation of violative residues in pigmeat. When normal pig ration supplemented with 40 mg/kg was fed to grower pigs for 10 days. The maximum residue concentration in these pigs was 0.09 ppm. This occurred in one kidney cortex and in one liver.

A second group of pigs were fed feed top dressed with chlortetracycline to provide a therapeutic dose of 20mg/kg daily for 10 days. When these pigs were killed violative residue concentrations (0.6 ppm in kidney ; 0.1 ppm in muscle) were detected only in carcases of pigs fed full therapeutic doses and killed without any withholding period.

The pen vacated by these pigs was immediately occupied by previously unexposed pigs. These were killed at 24 hour intervals after introduction. The maximum tissue concentration in the exposed pigs was 0.13 in the kidney cortex of one animal.

These studies indicate that chlortetracycline residues decline rapidly after the drug is removed from the feed, are not caused by the concentrations which normally occur through cross contamination in compounding and are also unlikely to arise from exposure to pens recently vacated by medicated pigs.

RECORDS FROM FARM INVESTIGATIONS

A total of 138 farm visits were completed following a positive test result in a randomly selected carcase. The disease reports from these farms emphasised the prime importance of respiratory conditions in all ages of pigs (Table 6).

Table 6. Diseases reported by producers during farm visits

Condition	Number of producers reporting		
	in finishers	in growers	in weaners
Pneumonia	25	11	13
Rhinitis	2	2	5
Coughing	3	2	0
Scours	3	2	16
Blood scour	4	3	1
Arthritis	2		
Mastitis	1		
Erysipelas	1		
Meningitis			2
No disease problems			

The information included in the reports indicates that where Chlortetracycline is incorporated in feed, the underlying condition in fatteners or growers, is most frequently pneumonia or coughing. On 90 of 138 farms the natural ventilation was boosted by various form of mechanical assistance. The atmosphere was considered to contain excess ammonia in 16 and to be stale in a further 12 of 119 farm reports. There was excess dust in 1 house and in 3 the temperature was reported as "too hot". These reports were usually exclusive.

During the investigations pigs on 63.3% of the farms were considered to be clean but on 36.7% they were reported to be dirty.

Water is provided on a large majority of farms from the mains supply (63%) and on others from a farm well (26.8%). Nipples are the most common terminals (93%) of the individual delivery systems.

Feed was bought from commercial compounders by 91% of the producers and 95% of these stored the bulk materials in a bulk bin, 5% obtained their supply in bags (81% of all producers used a single miller and 19% obtained supplies from more than one miller). The 16% who were home mixers also stored the finished material in bulk bins prior to feeding. A majority (49.6%) used dry feeding using a mixture of pelleted and non-pelleted meal, 42.6% fed wet and the remainder used both wet and dry feeding preparations. Almost all of the systems used the same pipeline or augers to deliver feed to the pens and in a number of cases the visiting officer reported that there was no facility for purging the delivery system after supplying medicated feed. Only 11 farms used floor feeding and 17 used a combination of floor and trough. The remainder (77.5%) supplied feed in some form of feeder. At the time of inspection 13% of these were found to contain residual quantities of feed.

Fifty-nine per cent of producers transported their own pigs to the plant, 37.6% used a commercial haulier and 3.4% used both means of transport. Approximately 70% of the pigs were supplied to the plants direct from the farm without mixing with pigs from another producer. The distances between 71 self haulier farms and plants were normally short (Table 7) and none of the pigs were involved in overnight transportation.

Table 7. Distance between farm and plant

Distance	Number of producers
<10	14
10 - 19	17
20 - 29	13
30 - 49	13
>50	14

SUMMARY

Chlortetracycline is the most frequently detected antibiotic residue in pig tissue. The frequency of detection has remained relatively constant. When therapeutic concentrations were fed to grower pigs violative residue concentrations were detected only in carcases of pigs killed without any withholding period. By 48 hours muscle and kidney concentration had shown a tenfold decline and was less than 50% of the MRL. It is therefore highly improbable that the residue violations are due to persistence following properly administered therapy.

Contamination of the environment of pigs by the excreta of medicated pigs can cause detectable concentrations in the tissues of previously clean pigs. However these do not approach the maximum permitted residue level at any stage up to 48 hours of exposure. As they are declining after this interval it is highly unlikely that the violations observed in the pig residue control scheme are due to contamination occurring either from contaminated pens on farms or in lairages.

As violative concentrations of chlortetracycline are unlikely to be caused by cross-contamination at the concentrations normally detected in feeds. Nor are they likely to arise from direct contact medicated and unmedicated pigs or from exposure of unmedicated pigs to the excreta of medicated pigs. It may be argued that the persistent level of violations arise from other sources the most probable of which is continued use of Chlortetracycline to control disease in fatteners on farms on which the feeding and management systems do not readily permit separation of medicated and unmedicated feed leading to slaughter weight pigs receiving medication close to slaughter. This area requires more detailed study.

SWINE VESICULAR DISEASE IN THE NETHERLANDS THE USE OF EPIDEMIOLOGY IN POLICY MAKING

W.J.H. VAN DER SANDE AND R.E. KOMIJN [1]

Swine Vesicular Disease (SVD) is an infectious viral disease in pigs. The disease is caused by an entero-virus. It is a very stable virus and able to survive for a long time in e.g. manure. The clinical symptoms are very similar to those of foot-and-mouth disease which is also the main reason why SVD is qualified as a List A disease and is therefore notifiable. Small quantities of virus in manure can infect the animals through skin lesions during transport or after arrival. The incubation time of SVD-virus can be very short. Experimental infections have shown that clinical symptoms can be seen in 2 days and antibodies can be detected 4 days after infection.

After an absence of 17 years Swine Vesicular Disease (SVD) was diagnosed on three farms in the central part of the Netherlands on July 1992. As a consequence of these three outbreaks, and the complaints by the Italian authorities that SVD had been found in pigs imported from the Netherlands, an extensive epidemiological survey was carried out. This paper gives a description of the methods used in this survey, the results and the effects on policy making with regard to SVD and pig health in general.

In November 1992 the EC concluded that the Netherlands was free from SVD, but again in February 1993 following Italian complaints of the presence of SVD in Dutch pigs the Netherlands was confronted with severe measures and restrictions. As a consequence the Netherlands developed a system in order to give farms of origin an "SVD-free" status.

When all measures were lifted in August 1993 the Dutch pig industry was unanimous in its wish to change the system into an overall monitoring/guarantee system in order to have a known health status for each pig holding in the Netherlands. A description of this monitoring system is given.

I. ClINICAL OUTBREAKS JULY 1992

On 4 July 1992 clinical symptoms of SVD were reported on a rearing farm (92/01) in the municipality of Ede in the centre of the Netherlands. The diagnosis was confirmed virologically and serologically at the ID-DLO Lelystad (the former CDI). All pigs were killed and destroyed. In the subsequent screening of the protection zone (3 km) all pig holdings were clinically inspected. Only contacts and suspect cases were serological screened.

[1] Veterinary Epidemiology Division, Veterinary Service, Ministry of Agriculture, Nature Management and Fisheries. P.O. box 20401, 2500 EK The Hague, The Netherlands.

A week later the rearing farm next door (92/02) reported clinical symptoms. On 27 July a screening team detected vesicles in a fattening herd (92/03) at a 500 meter distance from the first affected farm. In both cases the diagnosis was confirmed virologically and serologically.

No further outbreaks could be identified when the protection zone was screened and all contacts of the three outbreaks were traced. The imposed area restrictions were lifted on 13 August 1992. The restrictions on the export of live pigs, originating from this area, were lifted on 28 August 1992.

II. EXPORT PROBLEMS 1992 WITHOUT CLINICAL OUTBREAKS IN THE NETHERLANDS

On 3 September 1992 the Italian authorities reported clinical symptoms of SVD in a Dutch consignment of fattening pigs. SVD-virus was isolated and antibodies were found at the laboratory in Brescia (I). All 33 Dutch farms of origin related to this consignment were located within a 50 km radius of the three outbreaks of July. Therefore, a complete standstill of pigs came into force in this area on 8 September which from now we shall call "the restricted area".

On 12 September 1992 Italy reported positive serology and virology for SVD in another consignment with fattening pigs imported from the Netherlands. This time 194 Dutch pigs originating from 72 holdings were involved, of which 18 were located in the restricted area mentioned above. As the other 54 farms were located all over the Netherlands, national control measures were taken such as a total export ban of pigs and closing of markets, auctions and shows involving pigs.

Positive serology has been found in three more consignments with pigs originating from the Netherlands, concerning two consignments to Italy (one with piglets, the other with fattening pigs) and one to Belgium (piglets). These facts indicated that the Netherlands had a serious SVD problem. Therefore an extensive epidemiological survey was started in this area.

Material and methods for the epidemiological survey 1992

Starting point for the epidemiological survey were the concrete facts.

- There had been three SVD outbreaks very close to each other in Ede situated in the central part of the country.
- SVD had been diagnosed in pigs on a number of transports to Italy and Belgium.
- No further outbreaks were reported.

There are two ways to investigate the spread of the disease and possible outbreaks. Tracing the farms of origin of suspected/infected animals and their contacts is one way. Screening of a population at risk is an other. Both ways were used in this epidemiological survey.

Tracing: The farms of origin involved in the transports mentioned were traced. All the farms were clinically and serological investigated. The blood sampling was based on an expected prevalence of 5% at 95% confidence-level (reference Mrs. Owen, MAFF, UK). Fattening pigs are usually kept in pens (10 animals per pen). Because of the fact that SVD spreads very fast within one pen, fattening farms were sampled at a level of 1 pig per pen with a maximum of 60 blood samples. When no pigs were present because all of them had been sold important contacts were traced and clinically and serologically investigated.

In addition all contacts of the three former outbreaks were inspected again and blood samples were taken.

Screening: In the Netherlands there are 15 million pigs at approximately 28,000 pig holdings. Screening of the entire population is therefore too laborious and time consuming. Almost 50% of the farms of origin involved in the first 2 transports to Italy were located within a 50 km radius of the three outbreaks in Ede. If the infection was a regional problem, more outbreaks were to be expected in this area (the restricted area). Therefore, the screening was limited to the restricted area. All pig holdings in the former protection zone around Ede (3 km) were clinically inspected and blood samples were taken on the same basis as used for tracing. In the surveillance zone around Ede (10 km) 50% of all holdings were investigated. In the rest of the restricted area all holdings with sows were investigated.

To prevent serious welfare problems due to overcrowding from 5-8-1992 on pigs ready for slaughter from the restricted area were allowed to be slaughtered under supervision of the authorities. The meat had to be sold for national consumption. At the three designated slaughterhouses from 10% of the pigs blood samples were taken.

For the entire operation of SVD-control more than 300 persons from different organisations were directly involved. The organisation scheme for SVD-control is in annex 1.

Results from the epidemiological survey

An infected breeding farm (92/04) and a collection centre (92/05) were confirmed on 25 September, following the screening project of the protection zone around Ede. These two holdings were located at a distance of only 500 meters from the first 3 outbreaks (92/01, 92/02, 92/03). The pigs on both locations had been thoroughly inspected several times in July and August and no clinical symptoms were found. Nor were any lesions found in September while a big percentage of the pigs were serologically positive. This high number of serologically positives suggested that these pigs had been infected some time before. Probably during the period of the first three outbreaks in that area.

Outbreak 92/06 was confirmed on 26 October 1992. This fattening farm was located in Putten in the restricted area at a distance of approximately 15 km from the other outbreaks and had been identified through sampling of slaughter pigs in the designated slaughterhouses. The owner had not seen any symptoms. At the inspection of the killed animals several old lesions were detected.

In the tracing projects 628 holdings were investigated and from 32,039 pigs blood samples were taken (50 pigs per holding on average). The total pig population at these holdings was 277,031 and could be considered as a population highly at risk due to contacts with the infected holdings/transports. All clinical inspections and results of the blood samples were negative. Therefore, this survey indicated with

95% confidence that prevalence of SVD in this highly at risk population was less than 0.01%.

A total of 68,019 blood samples from 2,634 pig holdings were taken.

Outside the restricted area pre-export clinical inspections were required on the basis of Commission Decision 92/478/EEC. 12,000 pig holdings were inspected and no clinical symptoms were found.

Discussion

The overall conclusion of the epidemiological survey was that the SVD problem was limited to a relatively small region in the central part of the Netherlands. This conclusion was strongly supported by the fact that:

a. all tracing projects showed negative results
b. clinical inspection of 12,000 pig holdings outside the restricted area showed negative results
c. the 3 new outbreaks were all situated in the restricted area, of which 92/04 and 92/05 were located very close to 92/01, 92/02 and 92/03. Outbreak 92/06 was located at a distance of 15 km from the others.

None of the farms of origin related to the transports to Italy and Belgium could be identified as infected with SVD. It was concluded that the pigs on these transports had not been infected on the farms of origin, but during transportation or even in Italy. It is known that SVD has been a problem in Italy for years.

However, it is very likely that transportation has played a very important part. Manure samples were taken from 2 pig transportation vehicles involved with the transport of pigs to and from 92/06. SVD-virus was found in both of them. Other transport vehicles were sampled as well, but all were negative. The importance of the transportation network is also illustrated by the tracing scheme in annex 2. This scheme shows that all outbreaks are somehow related to each other and to the transports to Italy and Belgium.

Although it is difficult to prove how the virus was introduced, there are strong indications that the outbreak 92/05 played a major part. Through its many international contacts the virus could have been introduced at this collection centre and spread to its four neighbours. It is not unlikely that the pig trade from this collection centre introduced small concentrations of SVD-virus in transportation vehicles. The presence of small concentrations of SVD-virus in manure particles in transportation vehicles may be an explanation for the fact that pigs transported to Italy could be infected while SVD was not present on the farms of origin.

As a result, very much attention is given to cleansing and disinfection of the transportvehicles and the collection centres. This has been laid down in national legislation.

The survey's results were presented to the Standing Veterinary Committee of the EEC and all restrictions for the Netherlands were lifted by the end of November 1992. At the request of the Committee over 2,000 blood samples were taken from sows at slaughterhouses. The results were all negative for SVD.

III. EXPORT PROBLEMS 1993 WITHOUT ANY OUTBREAKS IN THE NETHERLANDS

On 26 February 1993 again the Italian authorities reported SVD in pigs imported from the Netherlands. The EC reacted almost immediately and banned all export of live pigs from the Netherlands and Italy on 1 March 1993. There had been no outbreaks in the Netherlands after the last one on 26 October 1992 and tracing the farms of origin related to the transports to Italy showed negative results. The export ban lasted one month. In April export became possible again, but only after certain measures had been taken. Before export pigs had to be tested serologically with a negative result. In the Netherlands a special project team, consisting of representatives of the government and pig industry, was put together for the organisation. The basic idea of the EC was to take blood samples from 10% of the fattening pigs to be exported and from 100% of the breeding and production pigs. The Dutch project team suggested an alternative for the last category. The alternative was to give holdings with breeding and production pigs a "SVD-free" status, based on random blood sampling of the pig population (again expected prevalence 5%; 95% confidence-level). If the result of the serological test was negative, the pig holding got an "SVD-free" status for three months, which allowed the export of pigs for that period.

The Commission of the EC agreed on this alternative and the measures to take blood samples were laid down in Commission Decision 93/177/EEC. Within a short period the project team had to develop an organisation structure for the blood sampling programme.

The organisation of the blood sampling programme

The Regional Animal Health Services (RAHS) co-ordinated blood sampling on pig holdings. There are 4 RAHS-s in the Netherlands and they are independant institutes. They carry out animal health programmes and are paid partly by farmers, partly by agricultural organisations and partly by the government. The National Animal Health Committee is their umbrella organisation, who is responsible for the pogrammes and tasks financed by the government and agricultural organisations. The RAHS drew up an application form for pig holders to send back if they wanted to have an "SVD free status" or wanted to export fattening pigs. On the basis of the application forms the RAHS organized and planned visits by veterinary practitioners, who carried out the blood sampling. In the case of fattening pigs, the pigs sampled got a special ear tag with the unique farm number and the qualification "SVD '93". The veterinarian sent back the blood samples to the RAHS, which prepared them and sent them to the Central Veterinary Institute (ID-DLO) in Lelystad, the national reference-lab. If the results of the blood tests were negative, the pig holdings were put on a special "SVD-free" list. This list was important for the RAHS, but also for the National Inspection Service for Livestock and Meat (RVV), because of their responsibility for the export health certificates. Because of the fact that the RVV is also responsible for the execution of disease control in the case of outbreaks or suspicion of notifiable diseases, there was a RVV co-ordination team handling the completely computerized data. This team was responsible for the organisation of retesting SVD suspects.

In addition the European Commission decided that a screening had to be carried out of sows (5%) and boars (50%) at slaughterhouses in all Member-States. This screening was laid down in Commission Decision 93/178/EEC.

Results

In 4 months that these blood sampling measures were in force, over 300,000 blood samples were taken at apporoximately 13,000 pig holdings, which is about 40% of all pig holdings in the Netherlands. More than 5,000 holdings with breeding and production pigs got an "SVD free status", the other 8,000 holdings were involved either in blood sampling fattening pigs for export or in the screening of sows and boars at the slaughterhouse.

The serological test showed a small proportion of false positives, which were called singleton reactors. In the Netherlands the number of singleton reactors was between 0.1% and 0.2%. The screening of sows and boars, carried out in all Member-States, showed that a certain amount of singelton reactors were found in all Member-States. So far, there is no clear explanation, but other entero-viruses might be responsible for cross-reactions. However, real outbreaks of SVD could not be identified.

IV. GUARANTEE SYSTEM

In May 1993 the measures for fattening pigs were lifted by the EC, but the Dutch government and the Dutch pig industry decided to continue blood sampling for this category, using the system of "SVD free holdings". The decision was made because people were afraid that another report by the Italians of positive serological findings in Dutch pigs would lead to an export ban again. For the same reason the Dutch pig industry wanted to continue the system on a regular basis for all Dutch pig holdings when all EC measures ended in August 1993. The Dutch governement and Dutch pig industry agreed on changing the system of "SVD free holdings" into a National Pig Health Control Programme.

The National Pig Health Control Programme

The aim of the programme is to have a known health status for every pig holding in the Netherlands, which gives extra guarantees of being free from notifiable diseases like SVD and classical swine fever. With this programme the Dutch pig industry hopes to avoid export bans in the future. How does it work?

Every pig holding in the Netherlands is visited by a veterinarian every 4 months. During this visit the pig population is clinically inspected on notifibale diseases. In addition blood samples are taken and will be serologically tested for one of the notifiable diseases (only SVD at this moment). Sampling is based on a random sample (expected prevalence 25%, 95% confidence-level), which is a rather small sample size (12 blood samples per holding at maximum). However, assuming that the pig popultion is free from notifiable diseases and taking into account the combination of clinical inspection and blood sampling, the sample size will do as a surveillance system.

The veterinarian writes down his clinical findings on a form and sends it, together with the blood samples, to the Regional Animal Health Service (RAHS). The RAHS registers the findings per holding, prepares the blood samples and sends them to the Central Veterinary Institute, where they are tested serologically. If the results of both clinical inspection and serology are negative, the holding is given the status of "approved holding" for a period of 4 months.

It is laid down in legislation that only approved holdings are allowed to have pigs and to move pigs. All pig holdings are registered in the central data-base of the RAHS. Therefore, the RAHS knows the status of each holding. An approved holding gets special stickers with name, address, unique farm number and period of validity. Every time the holding moves pigs, the identification and registration (I&R) form has to be provided with one of these stickers and the ear tag numbers of the pigs. All pig movement has to be recorded in the books at the holding.

It is laid down in legislation also that pig traders, pig transporters, slaughterhouses and collection centres are only allowed to accept or to transport pigs coming from approved holdings. Therefore, they are only allowed to accept or to transport pigs accompanied by I&R forms provided with a sticker. Offending traders, transporters and pig holders will be fined a maximum 4,000 Dutch guilders. Offending pig holders are also forced to join the health programme and they will pay a much higher fee. Offending slaughterhouses and collection centres might lose their EC approval.

The National Pig Health Control Programme came into force on 1 December 1993. As a consequence all pig holdings had to be visited at least one time before that date, because it was laid down in legislation that on 1 December 1993 all holdings had to have a known health status. The visits started on 1 September 1993. On 1 December 95% of all pig holdings in the Netherlands had been visited. The other 5% were either holdings registered in the central data-base, although they had ceased business or holdings that were empty by the time they were visited. It can be concluded that the introduction of the National Pig Health Control Programme was quite successful.

Problems encountered

In the beginning there was the problem of a small percentage of dead pigs due to sampling. This problem was not seen in earlier blood sampling actions and it turned out that a number of pig holders had changed to a breed which is more stress-sensitive.To handle this problem veterinarians, less experienced in blood sampling pigs, were instructed and supported by the RAHS. Nevertheless, a discussion was started about the question if it would not be better to have blood samples taken at the slaughterhouse. There are some reasons for the decision not to choose for this option (yet):

1. the pig population, which will be exported, does not take part in the serological screening;
2. because of its contacts with pigs from other holdings in the transportation network, the pig might not be representative for the farm

of origin when sampled at the slaughterhouse;
3. sample size, related to the farm of origin, will be smaller when carried out at the slaughterhouse, especially in those cases when small numbers of pigs per holding are being slaughtered (e.g. culled sows);
4. the combination of clinical inspection and blood sampling at the farm of origin encourages the veterinarian to carry out the clinical inspection more seriously.

Another difficulty is pig movement control. To verify if everyone in the pig production-chain works in line with the National Pig Health Control Programme, the correct use of stickers has to be examined. Especially when pigs are moved from one holding to another it is hard to have a clear view. Control is carried out by random inspections of the book-keeping of pig holdings.

This problem will be solved when the new identification and registration system for pigs, that is being developed at this moment, will be ready. In this new system all pig movement will be recorded in a central automated data-base, using the "voice-response" technique.

Results and effects

From 1 September 1993 until 1 December 1993 25,336 pig holdings were visited and 297,948 blood samples were examined. About 1,000 pig holdings were visited in December, because of the fact that they had already been visited in July and August when the EC measures were still in force. Only 14 offenders could be identified. They were fined and forced to take part by the General Inspection Service of the Ministry of Agriculture, Nature Management and Fisheries.

Because of the fact that attention is given to clinical signs of notifiable diseases, this programme also helps to monitor the threat of classical swine fever (CSF) from Germany and Belgium. CSF is present in both countries.

Another effect of this programme is that the whole pig production-chain is made responsible for the guarantees relating to pig health. Every link in the production-chain gives health guarantees to the following. This helps to make the whole production-chain aware of health risks and is an encouragement to work properly.

The system of giving health guarantees from the farm of origin is completely in line with the EC directives concerning health certification. Border inspections ended when the internal market came into force on 1 January 1993. The exporting country has to give health guarantees to the importing country. The health guarantees given in the health certificate refer to the animals, which are exported, and to the farm of origin. In the Netherlands pigs are being exported from collection centres. Health certification by the National Inspection Service of Livestock and Meat (RVV) takes place there and they do not have a clear view about the health status of the farms of origin. The health guarantees concerning the farms of origin given by the programme provides this missing link in health certification.

Plans for the future

For the future the plan is to complete the programme in such a way that it can function as being an overall guarantee system in the pig production-chain. This means in the first place that the health status of the holding will be linked to the hygienic status and the presence of risk-factors for pig diseases. Therefore, a lot of work has to be done in the field of risk analysis and the defining of GMP-codes. When this combination functions, it will be possible to relate the frequency of pig health control visits to the level of farm management. In other words: if farm management and hygienic status are poor the number of blood samples per year will be high and therefore expensive. Good management leads to a low number of blood samples per year. The aim of this system is to stimulate pig holders to strive for good pig farming and a high level of pig health.

A similar system can be developed for approved traders, transporters and so on, to strive for a high hygiene level in the transportation network.

The blood sampling programme will be extended to other diseases, like classical swine fever and Aujeszky's Disease in order to have a more complete surveillance system. The system will have to be flexible, so that it will be possible to switch to another disease whenever the disease situation in the Netherlands or surrounding countries forms a threat for the national pig population.

Finally, it has to be studied if a similar programme is worth developing for cattle, poultry, sheep and goats.

Epilogue

The SVD situation in the Netherlands has shown that the use of several epidemiological techniques can be very valuable to support policy making. On the basis of the combination of a classical technique (tracing) and modern techniques (random sampling, risk analysis) a lot of information is gathered for decision making.

For the future monitoring and guarantee systems are most likely to become more and more important in order to safeguard free movement of animals and products. To come to an overall high animal health level the industry will have to take their own responsibility.

FURTHER READING

Batho H.L., Costelloe A. and Gonzalez E., 1993. Report on an animal health mission to The Netherlands in relation to Swine Vesicular Disease, 14-15 april 1993. EEC report VI/3441/93: 7 p.

Blood D.C. and Radostits O.M., Veterinary Medicine. Bailliere Tindall, London

Fraser C.M. and Mays A., 1986. The Merck Veterinary Manual. Merck & Co., Rahway NJ, USA

Martin S.W., Meek A.H. and Willeberg P., 1988. Veterinary Epidemiology, principles and methods. Iowa State University Press, Ames, Iowa USA, (1988): 343 p.

Mededelingen VD, 1993. Regeling Bedrijfscontrole Dierziekten, een regeling van en voor het bedrijfsleven. Tijdschrift voor Diergeneeskunde; 118(23): 788-790

Owen J., Udias B. and Veroeveren P, 1992. Report on an animal health mission to The Netherlands on 30.09 and 01.10.1992 in relation to Swine Vesicular Disease (SVD). EEC report October 1992, 10 p.

Smak J.A., 1993. Interne markt: Uitdaging of Challenge. In Diergeneeskundig Memorandum. Benelux Press, 40(1993)1-2, 80 p.

Terpstra C, 1992. Vesiculaire varkensziekte in Nederland. Tijdschrift voor Diergeneeskunde; 117:623-626

Watson W.A., 1981. Swine Vesicular Disease in Great britain. Can Vet; 22(1981): 195-200

ANNEX 1 Organisation scheme for SVD - control

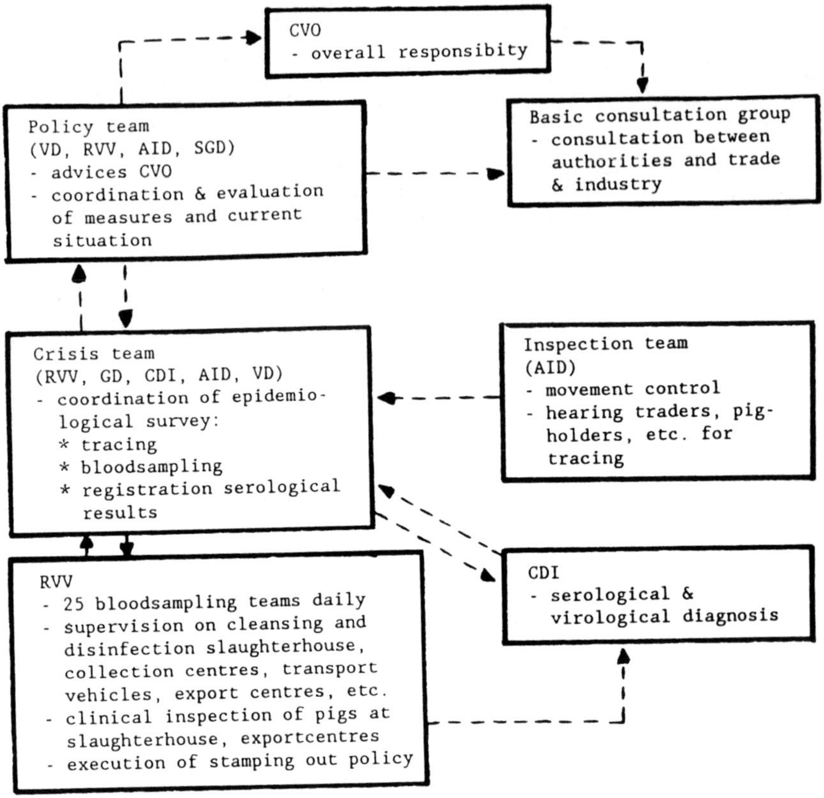

-------> = information line

VD	= Veterinary Service:	5 persons
RVV	= National Inspection Servive for Livestock and Meat:	± 250 persons
GD	= Regional Animal Health Service:	20 persons
AID	= General Inspection Service:	20 persons
CDI	= Central veterinary Institute:	15 persons
SGD	= National Animal Health Committee:	1 person

ANNEX 2

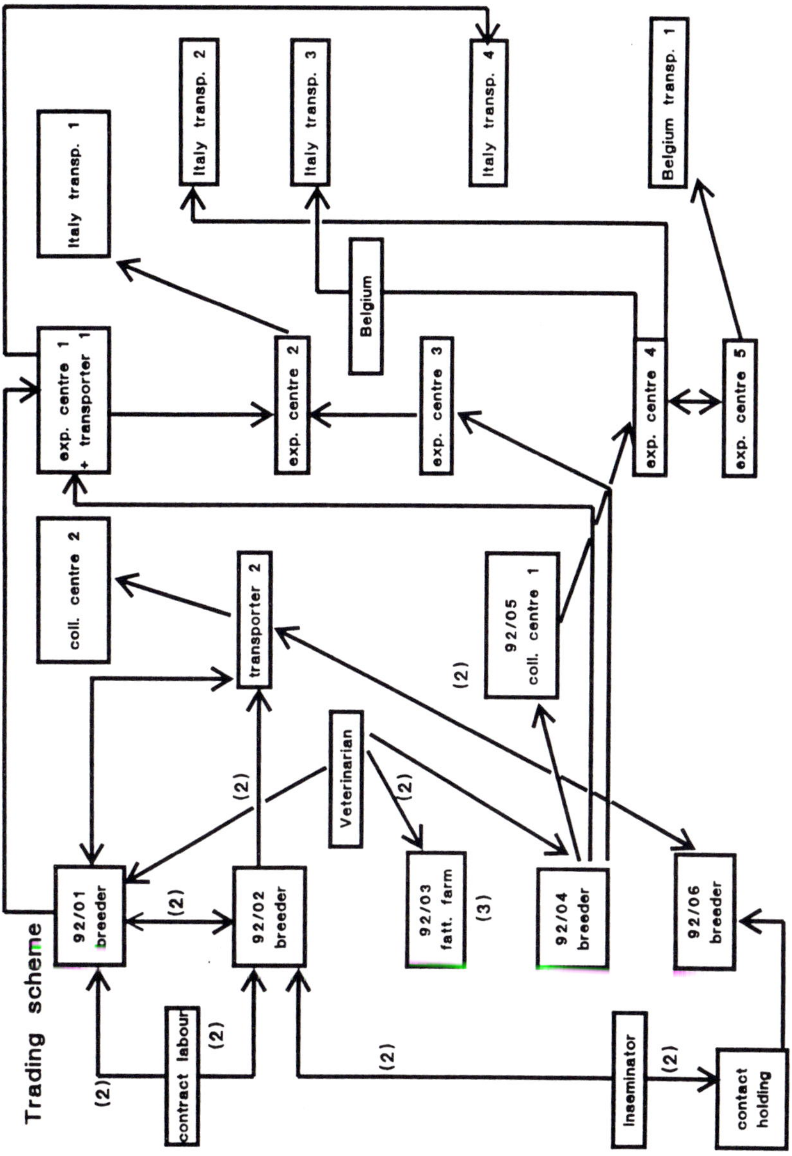

(2) = personal contacts
(3) = manure
ALL OTHER CONTACTS: ANIMAL MOVEMENT

ECONOMIC EVALUATION OF HOG CHOLERA IMPACT AND VACCINATION PROGRAMS IN HONDURAS BASED ON SMALL HOLDER SURVEYS

E. Hunt McCauley*

Hog cholera (HC) was first diagnosed in Honduras in 1952 and since then has prevailed to cause losses in spite of sporadic government vaccination initiatives. Small holder pig farmers in Honduras reportedly were suffering excessive HC death losses in the 1980's much like U.S. farmers suffered in the 1880-1915 era prior to the discovery and application of immunization techniques. Due to problems of vaccine availability and application to small holders' pigs, outbreaks were continuing to occur at unacceptable rates in Honduras. This study was undertaken to enable decision making about government investments in HC control programs and their returns to society.

The principal objective of this work was to determine the physical and financial dimensions of the impact of HC in Honduras and the possible control efforts for reducing this impact. Basic to this assessment was the determination of estimates of exposure probability, case incidence and clinical outcome of HC infection. In spite of recognized inaccuracies, owner surveys have been used in various situations as it has been the best method available for estimating the inefficiencies disease brings to livestock production (Heron & Suther, 1979; McCauley et al., 1983; Perry, 1983; Perry & McCauley, 1984). The owner survey described in this report was the only manner under Honduran conditions to collect production impact data required for this evaluation. This study deals exclusively with problems faced by small holder pig owners who raise about 90% of Honduras' pigs. The few larger, commercial producers usually having 20 or more sows carry out effective vaccination practices and were expected to continue this without public-sector assistance.

OWNER SURVEYS

Methods

Surveys were conducted by the author in the San Pedro Sula, La Ceiba, Tela and Choluteca areas. In each area some 15 owners were interviewed. These interviews were done in *municipios* simply by going from house to house asking about disease problems they had had with their pigs. Most were small holders with about 2 to 15 pigs of 3 to 15 months of age, including, in some cases, one sow which farrowed some 4 to 8 surviving piglets every year. Many pigs were *traspatio,* or roamed as scavengers by day and returned to the owners' premises at night. Owners were asked to describe their problems with HC *(el accidente)* which had occurred over the last 4-6 months.

*College of Veterinary Medicine, University of Minnesota, St. Paul, Minnesota 55108. Adjunct Faculty, Big Timber, Montana 59011.

Subsequently, Ministry of Natural Resources (MNR) officials conducted additional surveys in the San Pedro Sula (1,844 owners) and Choluteca (61 owners) areas. These surveys were conducted in accordance with guidelines developed during the author's surveys. In the Choluteca area only interviews of owners having problems with HC were reported. More HC problems had been recently reported from this area than from any other area in Honduras. The San Pedro Sula survey included interviews with owners having had recent HC problems as well as those who had not, and therefore yields more representative epidemiologic information.

Summary description of author's surveys

A diagnosis of HC as the cause of the problems reported by owners was based on signs reported of sudden onset of inappetence, conjunctivitis and copious lacrimation, severe abdominal respiration (*brinco*), severe depression (*morriña*), ataxia (*bolo* or *derrengado*) and death in 3-12 days. Reddened skin, shivering (*frio*) and huddling (*encimando*) were described in many cases. Diarrhea was usually reported, with hemorrhage in a few cases. Vomiting was reported by only two owners. A few owners described pigs being sick up to 30 days before they died.

Basically two pictures emerged: (1) HC had occurred in their community and death losses were 40 to 100% in unvaccinated and sometimes in vaccinated pigs. About 80% of the owners did not vaccinate. Several owners sold their apparently healthy pigs after a few pigs in their herd had died of the disease (called *el accidente*, *la morriña* and *el bolo*). In most cases owners reported that the disease had also occurred frequently in prior years. In these communities, owners were very interested in vaccination. Or, (2) In a few communities HC had not occurred for some time and they couldn't remember vaccinating in the past. These villages were usually remote with little traffic and poor road communication.

Survey findings by MNR officials

The results of owner surveys done by MNR officials in the San Pedro Sula and Choluteca areas are shown in Table 1.

The total (affected and unaffected premises) pig population of the samples in these two areas prior to recent problems with HC could not be determined in this survey. However, total pigs on hand at the time of the survey in the San Pedro Sula area survey done by MNR officials is an acceptable sample estimate as the population does not vary that much on the average and many owners who had lost pigs subsequently bought a few more. Accepting this, the mortality in the total population in the area sample for the recent four- to five-month period was 2,465/18,202 or 13.5%.[1] The probability of a premise being infected was indicated to be 21% (383/1,844). The interviewees said the average age of the pigs which died was 4 to 6 months and had an estimated value of $40/head. Pig owners surveyed in this area own more pigs (9.9 per owner) than the 4.9 per holding reported for small holders on the average for all of Honduras.

The surveys done by MNR officials were initiated by the author and agree basically with the findings of his numerous visits with owners in both areas. It is interesting to note

[1]An interesting comparison is that of a survey done in 14 countries in 14 states in the U.S. in 1912 and 1913 prior to the initiation of an immunization program. The annual mortality was 17.7% and 17.0% in the survey population in these years and dropped to 2.2% in the survey herds after an experimental immunization program was started in 1914. The sample population for each year was about one millions pigs (USDA/ARS, 1962). Another comparison is from the U.K. where it was concluded that the average mortality attributed to HC among all pigs on premises during HC outbreaks, including those born or moved during the quarantine period, was 20.4% (Ellis, 1972).

Table 1. Results of 1985 surveys of pig owners in *Municipios* of San Pedro Sula and Choluteca Areas of Honduras[a]

	San Pedro Sula[b]	Choluteca[c]
Number of *municipios*	9	6
Number of *aldeas*	195	20
Total owners interviewed	1844	61
Total pigs owned at time of interview	18,208	N.D.
Number owners with recent HC problems	383	61
Pigs on affected premises prior to HC, therefore presumably exposed	4,704	617
Deaths due to HC in presumably exposed pigs. Diagnosis based on history given.	2,465 (52.4%)	362 (58.5%)
Range of mortality in presumably exposed pigs (average per *municipio*)	29% to 89.5%	41% to 85%
Owners with HC problems who had vaccinated recently, in many cases after losses started	109 (28.5%)	12 (19.6%)
Range of percent of owners who vaccinated (averages per *municipio*)	0 to 38%	0 to 45%

[a] These surveys were initiated by the author and carried out by MNR officials over a 2-week period in March 1985.

[b] At the time of the interviews 1,461 owners (79%) holding 15,970 pigs reported no recent problems with HC and only 16.7% of these reported that they had vaccinated, presumably in the last year or so.

[c] The Choluteca area includes only owners who had had problems with HC since October 1984. In the San Pedro Sula area owners were interviewed regardless of whether or not they had had recent HC problems.

N.D. = not determined.

some similarities in these two survey results even though they were conducted by different officials in the two areas. Mortality in presumably exposed pigs was 52.43% and 58.6%; and 28.6% and 19.6% of the owners had vaccinated in San Pedro Sula and Choluteca areas respectively.

ECONOMIC EVALUATION

The production impact of hog cholera in Honduras

Production and price data come from four reports which are in general agreement (Damm, 1981; Maner, 1983; Umaña, 1985; Van de Wetering, 1983). Epidemiologic and economic coefficient estimates are assumed to be constant over the five-year period regardless of the number of pigs vaccinated or produced, i.e., every year there will be the same high or low estimates of pigs in which mortality is avoided and then later marketed for consumption depending on the scenario assumed.

Pig population: 530,000; 90% or 477,000 raised by small holders.
Pork production: 11.1 million kg carcass weight 1985.
Pork product yield is 50% of 55 kg pig slaughter weight.
Retail level price elasticity for pork: (-)1.18.
Pork retail price: 8.14 Lempira per kg in 1985. (One Lempira = $0.50)
Program costs also based on 1985 prices.

The estimated annual HC mortality of pigs raised by small holders in Honduras is based on estimates of annual probability of infection/clinical illness and case-fatality. There was no data, such as serologic evidence, on probability of infection. Based on the field observations, owner survey data and discussions with various animal health professionals in Honduras, this annual probability of infection/clinical illness is estimated to range from 15% to 30% of the 477,000 pigs owned by small holders (90% of the total pig population). The "case-fatality" rate is judged from the owner surveys as percent HC deaths in pigs presumably exposed and range from about 40% to 70%. In this evaluation it seems reasonable, therefore, to use the following high and low annual mortality estimates as bases for calculating the possible production improvement from avoiding mortality.

High possibility:	(0.30)(0.70) = 21% or 100,170 more pigs produced per year.
Low possibility:	(0.15)(0.40) = 6% or 28,620 more pigs produced per year.

Losses due to delayed growth in surviving pigs are not calculated in this study, since it is hard to defend increased production costs, mainly feed, for pigs which for the most part are scavengers. Another loss or cost to owners which occurs but is not estimated in this evaluation is the cost of medicine that is sometimes bought to treat pigs sick with HC.

It is assumed that the average pig weighs about 18 kg and is about 5 months old at the time of death. Actually there was wide variation found in ages of pigs dying of HC -- from weaner pigs of 5 kg to adults of 55 kg. In this study the HC loss is calculated to impact one year later in the form of loss of 55 kg live-weight animals marketed for slaughter. This approach is used to calculate a pork supply increase from improved HC control, which would result in lower prices for pork products to consumers.

Program costs

The annual program costs to government for the two programs are shown in Table 3. They were calculated from detailed costs for vaccines, salaries, equipment, supplies, vehicles, motorcycles, and operating expenses from data collected in Honduras. It was assumed that all equipment and vehicles were purchased in the program's first year (year 0). The costs are directly related to the major assumptions for vaccine coverage and the operational differences between the "intensive" and "owner participation" programs with the "owner participation" program costing the least due to the need for fewer personnel and vehicles and fewer doses of vaccine. Another important difference is that under the "owner participation" plan, owners would be required to purchase the vaccine from government teams visiting their villages. An estimated 80% vaccine cost recovery reduced the overall cost of this plan to the public sector. (The actual societal cost would include vaccine purchased). Since the threat of HC would be perceived differently in different communities based on their experience with HC problems, the purchases of vaccine per pig owner would vary considerably. Based on the field surveys this variation could range from 0% to 100% of pig owners wanting to purchase vaccine for their pigs. The vaccine coverage or usage is estimated at 60% for the "owner participation" program.

Benefits from hog cholera vaccination

Under the two programs, the reduction in losses is assumed to be 90% for the "intensive" program and 75% for the "owner-participation" program. There would be a greater reduction in mortality than indicated by vaccine coverage (percent of population vaccinated every year). With fewer animals susceptible, there would be fewer opportunities for virus multiplication in its natural host and therefore less dispersion to susceptible, unvaccinated pigs. This epidemiologic phenomenon is arbitrarily represented in the present study by estimating that, under the "intensive" program where 85% coverage is achieved, the reduction in mortality is estimated to be 90%. This same relationship is estimated for the "owner-participation" program but at a greater difference -- 75% reduction from a 60% vaccine coverage. This larger difference is meant to capture the nature of the "owner-participation" idea. Those owners having or seeing frequent problems with HC will undoubtedly buy and apply the vaccine at a higher rate and be rewarded with larger reductions in losses. So, it is argued that the "owner-participation" approach is more efficient through vaccine application in communities where the problems are the greatest.

Therefore, using the high and low mortality rates, the increased production of pigs which are assumed to be slaughtered one year later for consumption are:

"Intensive" Program	"Owner-Participation" Program
High losses: 100,170 pigs (90%) = 90,153	High losses: 100,170 pigs (75%) = 75,128
Low losses: 28,620 pigs (90%) = 25,758	Low losses: 28,620 pigs (75%) = 21,465

Accepting the assumptions of 55 kg slaughter weight per pig at marketing one year after mortality is avoided and 50% yield of pork product for retail marketing, the supply increase of pork for consumption and resulting incremental consumer surpluses are shown in Table 2. This is a "static" analysis in the sense that production is not assumed to change when lower prices are passed onto farmers. The estimated streams of benefits and costs and their discounted ratios are shown in Table 3.

Table 2. Annual benefits to Honduran consumers from losses avoided by hog cholera vaccination

Program	Mortality Avoided Estimates[a]	Increased Pigs (Head/year)	Increased Pork[b] (Million kg carcass/year)	Increase in Pork Supply (%)[c]	Decrease in Consumer Price (%)[d]	Incremental Consumer Surplus[e] (L million/year)
Intensive	High	90,153	2,459	22.3	18.7	18.738
	Low	25,758	709	6.4	5.4	5.040
Owner Participation	High	75,128	2,049	18.6	15.6	15.415
	Low	21,465	585	5.3	4.5	4.178

[a] For the "intensive" program, high is 90% reduction of a 21% mortality and low is a 90% reduction of a 6% mortality. For the "owner-participation" program, high is a 75% reduction of a 21% mortality and low is a 75% reduction of a 6% mortality.

[b] 55 kg slaughter weight one year later, 50% yield of pork product for retail market.

[c] 1985 pork carcass production is estimated to be 11.1 million kg. This may not include "back yard" slaughter.

[d] Using compensated direct price elasticity of (-)1.18 at the retail level for pork (Van de Wetering, 1983).

[e] This is the estimated incremental consumer surplus under these assumptions beginning the year following the program commencement and is assumed to continue at this annual level. One Lempira (L) = \$0.50. Based on 1985 retail price of L 8.14/kg; calculated by example:

$$(\Delta P)Q_o + \frac{1}{2}(\Delta P)\Delta Q = \left(\frac{L\ 1.52}{kg}\right)(11.1\ million\ kg) + \frac{1}{2}\left(\frac{L\ 1.52}{kg}\right)(2.46\ million\ kg) = 18.738\ million\ Lempira$$

Table 3. Benefit-cost values and ratios for hog cholera impact and vaccination control scenarios in Honduras

Program scenarios benefit assumptions	Year	End of year estimated benefits[a] to society (Million Lempira)	End of year estimated costs[a] to government (Million Lempira)	Ratio of benefit and cost present values[b]
"Intensive"	0	0	2.380	
21% mortality,	1	18.738	1.857	53.50 / 6.62 = 8.1
85% coverage and	2	18.738	1.857	
90% reduction	3	18.738	1.857	
	4	18.738	0	
"Intensive"	0	0	2.291	
6% mortality,	1	5.040	1.817	14.39 / 6.44 = 2.2
85% coverage and	2	5.040	1.817	
90% reduction	3	5.040	1.817	
	4	5.040	0	
"Owner Participation"	0	0	0.964[c]	
21% mortality,	1	15.415	0.680	44.01 / 2.52 = 17.5
60% coverage, and	2	15.415	0.680	
75% reduction	3	15.415	0.680	
	4	15.415	0	
"Owner Participation"	0	0	0.964[c]	
6% mortality,	1	4.178	0.676	11.93 / 2.51 = 4.7
60% coverage, and	2	4.178	0.676	
75% reduction	3	4.178	0.676	
	4	4.178	0	

[a] "End of year" means that costs or benefits are assumed to occur on December 31 of that year. This is to avoid calculations of essentially daily occurrences of disbursements or realization of benefits in order to annualize these values. December 31 of year zero is "day one" of the program and start of reduction in mortality. Benefits are calculated from savings consumers enjoy from increased pork supply from HC mortality reduction realized one year earlier. One Lempira = $0.50.

[b] Discount rate = 15% per year. The interest rate, charged by the Central Bank of Honduras to borrowers in their *Proyecto de Credito Agropecuario*, was 14.8% in March 1985. Internal rates of return were all well over 100%.

[c] The recovery of costs to government from the purchase of vaccine by owners is reflected in these costs. The total cost to society would actually be greater to include the purchase of vaccine by pig owners (about 304,000 Lempira per year) under the "owner-participation" program.

DISCUSSION

In evaluating financial consequences for any animal disease control program, one can derive a wide variety of b-c ratios depending mainly on the estimates of the losses caused by the disease and the efficacy of the control method. The evaluation in this study attempts to bracket high and low level loss potentials that can reasonably be defended from data available. These losses are weighed against the results of two potential control efforts, one "intensive" and more expensive compared to an "owner-participation" program characterized by less expense to government due to vaccine cost recovery but more efficiency at a lower level of vaccine coverage. This evaluation framework represents a range of reasonable possibilities. The "static" and "partial" nature of this analysis should be appreciated in that endogenous (production and consumption adjustments) and exogenous (population, income, foreign trade, etc.) factors have not been taken into account (Aulaqi and Sundquist, 1979). Another consideration regarding the b-c ratios is that this study treats HC losses in a conservative manner. It does not include growth delay or reproductive inefficiency (abortion, anestrous, etc.), which are also production losses from HC infection, but the incidence, time or occurrence and dimensions of these impacts are much more difficult to measure and defend than are those for death losses.

The b-c ratios estimated from analysis and data used indicate that either type of vaccination program is financially justifiable even at low levels of HC losses avoided. This benefit is measured as it affects pork consumers (Mishan 1975). Pig producers would realize increased total revenue since the quantity demanded by consumers increases more than the price decreases under conditions of the elastic price demand. The incremental producer surplus probably would be less than the incremental consumer surplus[2]. Revenue increases would be shared disproportionately. Those producers who avoided large losses due to HC would enjoy greater increases than those who had no HC losses.

However, some pig producers would probably respond to lower prices by decreasing production from what it otherwise would be. Under intensive production this response is fairly rapid, like a year or so, as the inputs (mainly feed) would be shifted to the next most profitable enterprise. This is not the case for traditional, scavenging pig production, so such a production response would be expected to be much less or slower than for intensive production. Certainly there would be fluctuating adjustments in both producers' and consumers' responses to improved efficiency in pig production, but the net effect of these fluctuations on the discounted benefits-and-cost relationships for the estimated scenarios is expected to be negligible over the five-year period.

Incremental consumer's surplus was used to value the increased production, as this was considered to best represent the value of benefits to society (Mishan, 1975). Some rather arbitrary assumptions were used in this approach in that this effect would remain stable over the years considered and that the price demand elasticity for pork would be constant over the increases in supply estimated. Actually, this elasticity would probably not remain constant over the range of supply increases estimated in this study. As the supply increases pass 10%, or so, the elasticity would start to decrease because consumers' preference for pork has a limit regardless

---

[2]In this evaluation, the supply and demand curve model was assumed to be linear with parallel shifts in the supply curve. Note that the sizes and changes (positive or negative) of producers surplus and revenues as well as consumers' surplus resulting from technologic production improvements depend on the shapes of the supply and demand curves, i.e., whether linear or convex, and on the way supply curve shifts occur, i.e., whether they are parallel, pivotal, convergent, divergent or some combination thereof as described by Miller et al., 1988.

of the price, and they will pay less than the (-)1.18 elasticity would indicate as supplies approach this limit. Therefore, under conditions of the high increase in supply in this study, the price decrease would probably be greater than the 18.7% calculated. The result of this would be an even greater consumer savings for these high levels of increased pork supply unless the excess supply were to be exported. Export demand for pork facing Honduras would be expected to be perfectly elastic.

There would be other unquantifiable benefits from improved HC control. The entire animal health infrastructure could be strengthened resulting in improved disease control for other diseases as well as HC in much the same way that HC, brucellosis and tuberculosis programs have assisted in strengthening overall animal disease control in many countries. A specific benefit of the reduction of incidence of HC infection is the facilitation of surveillance for African swine fever (ASF) (McCauley & Sundquist, 1979). With HC outbreaks occurring frequently, as they were in Honduras, there is always the rational apprehension that ASF may be the cause of illness observed and that such an infection may go unreported for some time. The possibility of clinical HC masking the presence of ASF would be lessened with the reduction in HC infection. Although the present study refers principally to small, traditional pig owners or rural households, larger commercial pig owners would also be benefitted greatly by decreased HC virus transmission and risk of introduction to their herds due to a larger number of immune pigs in the general population. Another benefit may come from potential exports of pork after domestic demand is satisfied in Honduras.

ACKNOWLEDGEMENTS

This study was done for the Government of Honduras and was funded by the U.S. Agency for International Development. I am grateful to officials of the Honduran Ministry of Natural Resources who collaborated in the owner surveys. I greatly appreciate the review and comment on this manuscript by Professor Willis Peterson of the University of Minnesota and the word processing and editorial assistance by Nancie Andersen of Big Timber, Montana.

REFERENCES

Aulaqi, N. and Sundquist, W.B. (1970). A Benefit Cost Analysis of Foot-and-Mouth Disease Spread and Control in the U.S. In E. H. McCauley, N. Aulaqi, J. C. New, W. B. Sundquist and W. M. Miller, Study of the Potential Economic Impact of Foot-and-Mouth Disease in the U.S., USDA Tech. Bulletin No. 1597, pp. 78-79.

Damm, J. (1981). Pork Production Development in Honduras. FAO report.

Ellis, P.R. (1972). An Economic Evaluation of the Swine Fever Eradication Programme in Great Britain. University of Reading, Dept. of Agriculture. Study No. 11. 76 pp.

Heron, B.R. and Suther, D.F. (1979). Survey of Incidence of Bovine Pulmonary Emphysema in California. Bovine Practitioner. 14: 1-8.

Maner, J.H. (1983). Small Farmer Swine Development Strategy for San Pedro Sula Region. USAID/Honduras report, International Agricultural Development Service. 69 pp.

McCauley, E.H. and Sundquist, W.B. (1979). Potential Economic Consequences of African Swine Fever and Its Control in the United States. Univ. of Minn., Dept. Ag. Econ. Staff Paper P79-11, 19 pp.

McCauley, E.H., Tayeb, A. and Majid, A.A. (1983). Owner Survey of Schistosomiasis Mortality in Sudanese Cattle. Tropical Animal Health and Production, 15: 227-233.

Miller, G.Y., Rosenblatt, J.M. and Hushak, L.J. (1988). The Effects of Supply Shifts on Producers' Surplus. American Journal of Agricultural Economics. 70-4:886-891.

Mishan, E.J. (1975). Economics for Social Decisions: Elements of Cost-Benefit Analysis. Measuring Consumers' Surplus. pp. 25-31. Praeger University Series U-747.

Perry, B.D. (1982). Owner Survey of Cattle Health and Production Factors in Zambia. FAO Document AG-DP/2AM/77/002.

Perry, B.D. and McCauley, E.H. (1984). Owner-Interview Surveys as a Basis for Estimating Animal Productivity and Disease Impact in Developing Countries. Proceedings Society Veterinary Epidemiology Preventative Medicine. Edinburgh, 54-62.

Umaña, E., O.J. (1985). Información Básica para el Proyecto Regional de Prevención Control y Eradicación del Cólera Porcina. OIRSA report.

USDA/ARS (1962). Supplement to the History of Hog Cholera Research in the U.S. in University of Minnesota Symposium on Hog Cholera. Edited by G. T. Mainwaring and D. K. Sorenson.

Van de Wetering, H. (1983). Macroeconomic Supply/Demand Analysis of Beef, Pork and Dairy Products in Honduras. Report to USAID/Honduras. 70 pp.

INVESTIGATION OF AN ACCIDENTAL RELEASE OF BACILLUS ANTHRACIS SPORES AT SVERDLOVSK

Martin Hugh-Jones

At about 6.30am on Monday, 2nd April, 1979 an accident occurred at the military biological research institute, "Compound #19", in Sverdlovsk, USSR. The nature of the accident is uncertain but it has been described by Soviet sources as an "explosion". As a result some 80 persons died of anthrax and 300-400 persons were hospitalised for treatment. Known human exposures were downwind of the institute and deaths occurred up to 4.4 kms from the institute. Domestic livestock (pigs, sheep and goats) and dogs died in the affected area of Sverdlovsk. The furthest direct cattle deaths from anthrax were 7 kms from the institute but sheep died up to 52 kms downwind and probably further. Present calculations indicate that between 1.0 and 50gms of B.anthracis spores were released in that single explosion using formulae based on single spore clouds.

Livestock Cases of Anthrax

There were sufficient dometic livestock deaths in Chkalovski Rayon in the southern sector of Sverdlovsk to result in door to door visits by the Oblast veterinary service. But their findings have not been published. Discussions with contemporary residents confirmed that there had been many deaths amoung domestic pigs and small ruminants and that some streets were affected, while others were not. In the 1988 meetings in the USA, General Burgasov claimed that dogs had died in Sverdlovsk; if correct, they could be from either large primary aerosol doses or from consuming fallen or butchered animals.

Some 17 people suffered from cutaneous lesions, six with toxaemia, and all recovered (Burgasov & Nikiforov, 1968 & 1988). It is claimed that all were a result of "occupational" exposures, eg skinning animals, (Cherkasskiy, pers com) but it is hard to explain all cutaneous lesions on this basis. One woman had a lesion on the nape of her neck and a man had a shoulder lesion, and another cutaneous case was said to have been the single child diagnosed with anthrax. The informal case lists kept by the Director of Hospital #24 have two notations of a dead goat and a sick pig in the Chkalovski Rayon. She stated during an interview thatthere were extensive small stock deaths in the Rayon cotemporaneous with the earliest human deaths. While we were given confusing statements of livestock deaths in early and late March, there

D/WHO Collaborating Center for Reference & Training in Remote Sensing and Geographic Information Systems for Veterinary Public Health, School of Veterinary Medicine, Louisiana State University, Baton Rouge, LA 70803, USA.

were authoritative statements from informed individuals that the livestock anthrax deaths did not preceed the human cases.

The various official and authoritative (eg General Burgasov, Prof. Ponomaryov) accounts gave ten settlements and villages outside Sverdlovsk affected with livestock anthrax. These lie on a straight narrow band at 330° from Compound #19. Ponomaryov recounted that a total of 68 isolations were made from animal cases with 60/68 involving privately owned animals from small holdings and the yards and gardens of private homes. In the outer villages there were instances of cattle dying but it was primarily of sheep and goats. These details were provided by General Burgasov and were copies of various contemporary documents acquired by the KGB. The objective was to persuade us that some or all of the human cases were in fact enteric anthrax, as a result of consuming infected animals; it is now known that all human deaths were from pneumonic anthrax. There is no reason at this time to believe that these documents were forgeries, though certainly selected.

The livestock events beyond the Chkalovskii Rayon are summarised in Table 1. Investigators searching for livestock deaths noted that a sheep had been illegally slaughtered and butchered in the village of Rudnyi on the 28th March; it was never checked for anthrax. The meat was sold to local people without ill effect. The same family slaughtered two more sheep on the 7th and 8th April and the three relatives dressing these carcases developed cutaneous anthrax. From the material provided this family had 2/5 sheep die from anthrax. T.A. Stafeyeta and her husband butchered a cow that had died during the night of 6/7th April and dumped the pieces into a pit; the investigators recovered two pieces of skin from this animal on 23rd April and it was Ascoli positive for anthrax. The Stafeyetas also butchered a six month old bull calf and a five month old piglet and sold the meat to five neighbours and relatives. While there is no record at this time of the latter animals being tested for anthrax, it must be suspected as it would not have made financial sense to kill and butcher animals so young.

Ears were collected on 6th April from three sheep belonging to three separate individuals in Kashino and examined for anthrax. The Sverdlovsk laboratory confirmed anthrax by culture in two on Sunday 8th April and noted that it was not possible to test the third as the veins were empty but that smears demonstrated "encapsulated microflora" similar to B.anthracis. This was the first diagnosis of anthrax in thisepidemic. "Encapsulated microflora" were also identified in an ear from a dead lamb in Pervomayskyi on the 12th April; the sample collection date is not stated but was presumeably on the 9th or 10th, if not significantly earlier.

On 22nd April the Sverdlovsk veterinary laboratory received some sausage confiscated in the Central Market, Sverdlovsk; the species involved were not given. The sausage meat were positive to the "hot precipitation method" and the rib meat negative. The specific origin of this material was not given.

Table 1:

REPORTS OF LIVSTOCK ANTHRAX RELATED CASES (Veterinariya (10)pp3-5 (1980); PN Burgasov documents; DN Ponomaryov, pers. com.)

Place	kms	April, 1979 2	3	4	5	6	7	8	9	10	11	12
Rudnyi	7	*	.	.	.	B	S	P S B	.	.	.	.
Bolshoye sedel'nikovo	16	*	no information available									
Maleye sedel'nikovo	17	*	no information available									
Pervomayskyi	23	*	one lamb diagnosed, report dated 12 April									
Kashino	32	*	.	.	.	S S S	.	.	.	.	.	.
Sysert	34	*	no information available									
Abramovo	52	*	.	.	S S	S S	S S	S	.	P B B B B	B	.

Notes:

B = bovine
P = pig
S = sheep

Laboratory confirmed anthrax deaths are underlined; effectively all tissues collected and submitted to the veterinary laboratory in Sverdlovsk demonstrated B.anthracis or B.anthracis-like organisms.

The most complete reports were from the outbreak in Abramovo On 22nd April the Sverdlovsk veterinary laboratory received some sausage filling and two ribs with attached muscles and the surrounding area; the first, a handwritten report, is dated the 13th April and the second typewritten report, incorporating the first with corrections, is dated the 25th April. Seven sheep from separate addresses became ill and/or died between the 5th and 8th April; anthrax was confirmed in 6/7, one on 23.4.79. On the 10th and 11th April five cattle and a pig were ill and/or dying, one at the collective farm in Averino; anthrax was confirmed in one yearling heifer. On Tuesday, 10th April, 1019 cattle on the Abramovo state farm (Sovhoz) were vaccinated with STI vaccine. By nightfall on the 11th a total of 1686 head - 1143 cattle, 125 sheep, 5 goats, 86 pigs, and 57 horses - had been vaccinated in Abramovo with STI and GNKI vaccines, and 325 animals, presumeably within the village of Abramovo itself, - 91 cattle, 173 sheep, 10 goats, 42 pigs, 3 horses - had received antiserum. This represents a significant logistic effort that would have necessitated a number of days to organise. Unfortunately it has not been possible to determine when it was ordered.

An extensive cleanup was then initiated on all affected establishments. The stable floor boards were taken up and burnt in a pit in the forest, and the underlying soil removed to a depth of 20cms, disinfected with 20% chlorine solution, and also dumped in the same pit 2 kms away. The affected yards were washerd down four times with 10% hot caustic soda and a final fifth time with a 0.1% solution of chlorophos. On 21.4.79 the cattle and horses receiving antiserum were vaccinated with STI vaccine and the small ruminants and pigs received GNKI vaccine. Other than two lambs dying from mauling and trampling by cattle there were no more deaths and quarantine was requested to be lifted on 25th April.

These livestock cases revealed a number of interesting facets of this outbreak. Firstly, it is clear that sheep are markedly more susceptible to airborne anthrax than cattle. From evidence presented to us in Yekaterinburg, it is possible that Compound #19 was using sheep as experimental animals and therefore one may not be surprised by such a sensitivity. It can be argued that the cattle and piglet ill in Abramovo might have been secondary cases, but this can only be confirmed or denied by further interviews, which we were denied. Secondly, it has not been possible to name all ten villages affected downwind. There is anecdotal evidence for a livestock case in Averino, 58 kms, from Compound #19. The proximity of other villages suggests that livestock deaths may have occurred 60 kms or more downwind. Thirdly, the absence of human cases beyond the Chkalovski Rayon in Sverdlovsk may be a function of exposure dose. On the other hand, the narrowness of the plume, both in the villages named and in mathematical model runs, indicates a very limited exposure. On the morning of 2nd April there was a 4-6m/sec wind, an air temperature around -5°C, and stable meteorological conditions. Outside activities in agricultural communities are always limited in winter-time and one must doubt that any villagers were dawdling outside after feeding their stock.

Lastly, the Oblast veterinarians were "on the ball". Not only did they diagnose the disease days before before this was achieved for the human deaths, which were initially being ascribed to "viral pneumonia", but their prompt response, as described for Abramovo, is impressive. What happened in the other villages to limit this epidemic awaits discovery.

Some Aspects of the Human Cases

Exactly how many humans died of anthrax is uncertain. The early, hyperacute deaths were misdiagnosed and not entered into the record. With the origin inside a military research institute, the apparent absence of military deaths must pose questions. The working estimate is that there were probably 80 deaths from anthrax. Surviving records show that that by the 20th April there was a total of 45 deaths, 214 patients were in Hospital #40 set aside specifically for clinically suspect anthrax cases, and 358 patients had been seen in outpatient clinics. Deaths, and presumeably surviving clinical cases, continued to occur sporadically until late May and the last death was on or about June 10th; the latter was a vagrant who was found dead. In the general population there was a widespread consumption of oral antibiotics. Human vaccination started on 21st April. Some 47,231 individuals were vaccinated one or more times with the Tblisi vaccine, with 1574 (3.3%) being later excused work because of the severity of side effects from the vaccine. The number of people affected was therefore some number less than five hundred, possibly in the range of 300 to 400.

Plotting the known cases using a GIS database based on a GPS registered SPOT image of the city, indicates a clustering of cases, and especially deaths, at 900m intervals from the probable source. This suggests that some form of leewave phenomenon may have occurred.

A puzzling aspect of the epidemic is the absence of cases amoung infants, children, teenagers and young adults; the few exceptions of named sick teenagers and university students only confirms this extraordinary absence. One can argue that there was either some form of age protection or that they were merely not outside to be exposed at the time the plume passed. While the median age of men dying (42 - 40 years) did not change between the two halves of the epidemic, the median age for women dying in the first half was 67 years (17) compared to 57 years (3) later. The necropsy records of 42 pathology confirmed anthrax deaths show that 19 had chronic lung lesions of one form or another - "welders lung" (8), centroasinar emphysema (8) and miscellaneous chronic lesions (9) with a number having dual conditions (J. Smith & L. Grinsberg, pers com). But without denominator rates for such conditions in the Rayon community, the frequency cannot be interpreted.

The time that the material was released may be estimated as follows. The 4-6 m/sec wind would have taken just under three hours to reach Abramovo. Because of increasing instability, it would have to have arrived before midday/early afternoon.

Therefore, the release had to be before 9.00am - 10.00am. Of all the people known to be ill working at the Ceramics Factory, which was directly in the downwind plume, only two were on the night shift; all others were on the 8.00am to 4.00pm day shift. This factory produces industrial ceramics, such as pipes and tiles. Thus, the night shift workers would have bgun to leave the plant sometime around 7.55am and many would have walked home as they lived in the Rayon. Therefore one might presume an absence of exposure between 7.55am and 8.30am. School started at 8.00am and therefore children and teenagers would have been in the nearby streets walking to school from 7.45am. The area Kindergarten (#385) was right in the midline of the plume and its teacher did die of anthrax; she also lived in the plume and was known to shower at the Ceramics Factory. While one might argue that the kindergarten itself might have been safe by being in a "skip" zone of the plume, but some of the mothers bringing their infants would certainly have walked through high risk areas if the plume was active at that time. Also we cannot assume that all those mothers were late teenagers or in their robust, healthy early twenties. Knowing the starting times for the various factories and work sites it is possible to trace the probable movements of individuals going to work that either lived on the edge of the plume, or moved into it, or crossed it. These movements indicate two exposure periods of 6.30am to 6.50am and from around 7.30am to 7.50am; this reflects the intense activity associated with day shifts starting at 7.00am and 8.00am. One individual lived inside the plume and had to leave home between 7.05am and 7.20am to get to work by 7.30am. Overall there is the probability that exposure occurred between 6.30am and 7.40am. This presumes that there was a "heat island" effect protecting the night shift workers in the Ceramics Factory and that the day shift was infected on the way to work or as they entered through the plant gate.

The alternative is that it happened shortly after 8.30am to account for the two night shift workers at the Ceramics Factory. This implies that there was no "heat island" to lift the plume over the plant, thereby exposing the day shift, and that all the traced individuals were late going to work at other sites that Monday.

Conclusions

The ongoing analysis of this epidemic has raised a number of questions of immediate relevance to the behaviour of infective aerosols, and specifically anthrax spores. There is an an almost total absence of information on the LD50 needed to kill sheep and cattle with an aerosol of anthrax spores; the frequency of lambs dying is of special interest. But they can act as competant sentinels for human exposure. The coincident porcine deaths suggest that secondary spread must be considered in two villages with implications for the interpretation of late bovine deaths. There was a difference in the bearing for the long distance sheep deaths (330°) and the short distance human deaths (340°). Present calculations indicate that 50gms of single-spore equivalents may be needed to kill sheep at

>50kms but about one gram for the human deaths. This suggests that the initial release had a vertical primary component into the undisturbed air stream and that the people were exposed to the residual secondary material following the "explosion" as the air passed over and through the built up area next to Compound #19.

THE EPIDEMIOLOGICAL SIGNIFICANCE OF FOOT AND MOUTH DISEASE VIRUS CARRIERS - A REVIEW

J S SALT[*]

Foot and Mouth Disease (FMD) is a highly contagious vesicular disease of even-toed ungulates, both domesticated and wild. It is caused by small single-stranded RNA viruses of the picornavirus family. The disease was first described in the Europe of the Middle Ages by Fracastorius in 1546, and remains a disease of world-wide economic importance today. FMD was the first animal disease shown to be caused by a virus (Loeffler and Frosch, 1898) and was only the second virus in history to be discovered.

The symptoms of FMD are those of an acute febrile illness accompanied by the variable occurrence of epithelial vesicles particularly at sites of trauma and epithelial hypertrophy, namely the mouth, feet, rumen and teats. In sheep and goats the disease is often less clinically severe than in cattle, making diagnosis more difficult in the field (Burrows, 1968; Pay, 1988). Different strains of Foot and Mouth Disease Virus (FMDV) show variable virulence within a species and differences exist in the virulence of individual virus strains for the various host species. Fatalities occur mainly in young animals due to myocarditis with some strains of the virus, although the major economic losses associated with FMD accrue from loss of production and the indirect cost of vaccination/control strategies, and interference with international trade. Chronic sequelae to FMDV infection have been recorded. These are associated with the initial damage to glandular tissues during the acute stages of infection and virus multiplication in internal organs, in particular involvement of the pituitary and thyroid glands results in the occurence of '*hairy panters*' in the Tropics.

Persistent infection is a common sequel to both clinical and subclinical FMD. Subclinical infection more frequently follows challenge with low titres of FMDV (Sutmoller et al, 1968) and in cattle with partial immunity. These conditions are thought to prevail in FMD endemic areas where animals are sporadically exposed to virus and maintain low levels of antibody to FMDV. In these animals virus replication occurs at primary sites in the oropharynx, but generalised disease is prevented by humoral antibody. This is also the case for FMDV vaccinated, protected animals where virus replication is again restricted to the oropharynx.

[*] AFRC Institute for Animal Health, Epidemiology Dept., Pirbright Laboratory, Ash Road, Pirbright, Woking, Surrey GU24 0NF, UK.

EPIDEMIOLOGY OF FMD

FMDV infection of susceptible animals in the field occurs primarily via the upper respiratory tract by inhalation of airborne virus from an infected animal (Donaldson, 1987), and occasionally in calves by insufflation of infected milk. The incubation period and susceptibility to FMD is dependent upon the dose and strain of virus, the species of animal, the route of infection and the level of existing immunity. Cattle are the most susceptible of the domesticated species to FMDV, as little as 10 tissue culture infectious doses are required to establish infection by inhalation. Higher titres of virus are required in all species to cause FMD by ingestion (Donaldson et al, 1987), pigs being more susceptible to FMDV infection by this route than ruminants. Infection is also possible through the skin from local trauma/abrasions, as occurs in the mammary gland of milking cows (Burrows et al, 1971) and the feet and legs in pigs.

The primary mode of transmission of FMDV during an outbreak is direct contact with a diseased animal. Secondary modes of transmission include contact with infected animal products and fomites, wind-borne spread, and mechanical transmission by vehicles and people. However, several reports of field outbreaks of FMD early in this century led to the belief that convalescent cattle may be responsible for the infection of susceptible in-contact animals. This appeared to be the case following the 1922-24 epidemic in the UK (Hedger and Stubbins, 1971), and was thought to explain the introduction and perpetuation of FMD in Mexico following the importation of cattle from Brazil in the 1940's (van Bekkum, 1973). However, evidence to refute the theory was also available from field observations (Mohler, 1926) and the many failed attempts to transmit FMDV from convalescent cattle under controlled experimental conditions.

Nevertheless, an unsubstantiated report by Waldemann et al in 1931, maintained that virus was present for several months in the urine of cattle after recovery from acute FMD. In 1959 van Bekkum et al reported the recovery of tissue culture infectious FMDV in oropharyngeal scrapings from FMD convalescent experimental cattle. This discovery irrefutably confirmed the existence of the FMDV carrier state and demonstrated that FMDV could establish a persistent asymptomatic infection in the upper respiratory tract of cattle. Subsequently, the natural occurrence of FMDV carriers was established by Sutmoller and Gaggero (1965) who described the recovery of FMDV in oropharyngeal fluid samples over prolonged periods following a field outbreak of FMD in cattle in Brazil.

THE CARRIER STATE IN FMD

A carrier of FMDV is defined as an animal from which FMDV can be recovered in oropharyngeal fluid samples using a probang sampling cup for periods of greater than 28 days post-challenge (Sutmoller et al, 1968). The oropharynx, and more particularly the dorsal soft palate, was suggested by Burrows (1966) and van Bekkum et al (1966) to be the predilection site for FMDV persistence in cattle, although infectious virus has been recovered for shorter periods from a number of organs and tissues during convalescence (Cottral, 1969). In carrier sheep however, the tonsillar region was found to be the site of highest titre and most frequent virus recovery (Burrows, 1968).

The titre of infectious virus in probang samples, as determined by tissue culture, is invariably low and gradually declines during the period of FMDV persistence (van Bekkum et al, 1966), to fall below the level thought to be necessary for successful transmission to susceptible animals (Donaldson and Kitching, 1989). The decline in titre and frequency of infectious virus recovery from the oropharynx may be accompanied by the increased production of non-infectious virus particles. Using the polymerase chain reaction (PCR) and dot-blot hybridisation, FMDV RNA fragments have been detected in probang fluid samples after infectious virus can no longer be isolated (Rossi et al, 1988). How these results relate to infectivity is not currently understood.

The duration of the carrier state is breed and species-related, inasmuch as different breeds of African cattle have been shown to excrete FMDV for up to 2.5 (Hedger, 1968) and 3 years (Hargreaves et al, submitted for publication), sheep and goats for up to 9 months (Burrows, 1968; Pay, 1988) and African Buffalo for at least 5 years (Condy et al, 1985). Strain variation also affects the capacity of FMDV to establish persistent infections. The S.A.T. serotype viruses are only able to maintain themselves in Africa, where there is a resident buffalo population which it has been suggested could act as a reservoir of infection.

In both vaccinated and non-vaccinated cattle the establishment of the carrier state occurs frequently following FMDV challenge, estimated at approximately 50% by Sutmoller and Gaggero (1965) 6 months after an FMD outbreak in Brazil. Experimentally this figure is even higher, presumably because of improved FMDV detection rates under laboratory conditions (Sutmoller et al, 1968) (see Table 1). Anderson et al (1976) found very few carrier sheep or goats in a field survey of an endemic area of Kenya, which led them to conclude that these animals did not play a significant role in the spread of FMDV in that country. Field evidence also shows that routine vaccination of cattle reduces the establishment of carriers in endemic areas (Anderson et al, 1974), probably indirectly by increasing herd immunity, thereby reducing the number of new clinical cases and thus challenge doses of FMDV.

EPIDEMIOLOGICAL IMPORTANCE OF FMDV CARRIERS

Transmission of FMDV from carriers

Auge de Mello et al (1966) showed that an attenuated, live lapinised FMDV vaccine strain would also transmit from vaccinated to susceptible cattle. However, the evidence for transmission of clinical FMD to susceptible animals from true FMDV carriers is circumstantial. Field evidence suggests that transmission occurs from carrier buffalo in Africa both to buffalo calves (Condy et al, 1985; Bengis et al, 1986) and to cattle (Hedger, 1970; Hedger and Condy, 1985). However, in FMD endemic areas it has been difficult to confirm carrier animals as the unequivocal source of further outbreak virus due to the problems presented by poor movement records, the number of outbreaks and precise identification of FMDV outbreak strains.

Table 1. Virus isolations on bovine thyroid cells from probang samples collected from cattle challenged with FMDV type O_1.

	Animal number						
Days p-i	RV17	RV18	RV19	RV20	RV21	RV34	RV35
0	-[a]	-	-	-	-	-	-
21	+[b]	+	-	nd	-	nd	nd
28	nd[c]	nd	nd	-	nd	+	
35	-	-	NT[d]	+	-	+	-
42	nd	nd	nd	+	nd	-	+
49	nd	nd	nd	+	nd	-	-
56	nd	nd	nd	+	nd	-	-
63	-	+	NT	+	NT	+	+
70	-	+	NT	+	-	+	+
77	-	+	-	+	-	+	+
84	-	-	-	+	-	-	+
91	-	-	NT	nd	-	nd	nd
98	-	-	NT	+	-	+	-
105	-	+	NT	+	-	-	-
112	-	-	NT	-	-	-	-
119	-	-	NT	nd	-	nd	nd
126	nd	nd	nd	+	nd	NT	-
133	-	-	-	+	-	+	-
140	-	-	NT	+	NT	+	-
147	-	-	-	+	-	-	NT
161	-	NT	-	-	-	+	-
168	-	NT	NT	nd	-	nd	nd
175	-	-	-	+	-	-	-
182	-	-	-	nd	-	nd	nd
196	-	-	NT	nd	NT	-	-
210	-	-	-	nd	NT	nd	nd

[a]-, negative c.p.e. after 72 hours
[b]+, positive c.p.e., positive for type O FMDV
[c]nd, not done
[d]NT, positive c.p.e., negative for type O FMDV

Despite reports of the seroconversion (van Bekkum et al, 1959) and isolation of pharyngeal FMDV from calves with carrier dams (Hedger, 1968), transmission of FMD from carrier cattle to susceptible animals has not been shown under controlled conditions. Several observations have been proposed to explain why the demonstration of transmission from FMDV carriers has been so elusive. These include the small numbers of animals inevitably used in transmission studies, the low virus titre in the oropharynx, the possible cell-association of persistent virus, the presence of neutralising antibody in secretory fluids, the dilution and swallowing of secreted virus in saliva and altered virulence/infectivity of carrier virus. However, the overall conclusion from these studies is that certain *stress factors*, as yet to be identified, are involved in the successful transmission of FMDV from carrier to susceptible animals.

In vitro work with a baby hamster kidney cell line persistently infected with FMDV has shown that attenuation of virus pathogenicity for both cattle and mice had occurred during co-culture and that this correlated with increased temperature and pH sensitivity and small plaque formation (Diez et al, 1990). Kaaden et al (1975) showed that carrier virus isolated from cattle was less cytopathic in cell culture than wild-type virus and showed reduced virulence for susceptible cattle. However, the carrier virus retained its virulence for pigs and guinea pigs, and regained its virulence for cattle after a single passage in pigs. Therefore, attenuation seems to be species or cell-type dependent and reversible in nature, as was found in the field when lapinised live FMDV vaccines were used.

Molecular epidemiology

The difficulties associated with tracing cattle movements and obtaining accurate disease reports from FMDV endemic areas have hampered the epidemiological investigation of the role of carriers in field outbreaks. However, recent developments in rapid nucleotide sequencing have allowed accurate identification and comparison of FMDV field isolates. The application of these molecular epidemiological techniques has been fruitfully applied in a collaborative ODA sponsored project between the World Reference Laboratory for FMD and Zimbabwe. These studies have demonstrated the long-term stability of carrier virus isolates, and has provided the most convincing evidence so far recorded for the role of FMDV carrier cattle in the initiation of field outbreaks of FMD (N.J.Knowles, unpublished data).

Certain unique features of the FMD situation in Zimbabwe have contributed to the successful molecular epidemiological studies in that country. These features include the low number of outbreaks, the high standard of animal movement control and record keeping, good disease surveillance and reporting, and the maintenance of a large central FMD-free region from which export to the E.C. is permitted. For the purposes of FMD control Zimbabwe is divided into four zones (Anderson et al, 1993). In the wildlife zone around the borders of the country FMD is endemic and is thought to be maintained by African Buffalo, which have been shown to be long-term carriers of all three S.A.T. serotypes of FMDV. The red zone is separated from the wildlife zone by a game fence and contains domesticated cattle which are vaccinated twice yearly against FMD. Green zones are fenced off from the red zones and contain non-vaccinated sentinel cattle, which are serologically tested for evidence of FMD prior to movement. The central clear zone is a designated 'FMD-free' region in which vaccination is not practised and from part of which export of cattle to the E.C. is permitted.

The molecular epidemiological investigation of FMDV field isolates from Zimbabwe has demonstrated two basic patterns of FMDV epidemiology. S.A.T 1 and 3 viruses appear to be maintained in African Buffalo populations, with sporadic short-lived outbreaks occurring in local cattle. Whereas S.A.T. 2 viruses appear to be maintained within the cattle population and have spread more extensively. It is the study of recent S.A.T. 2 FMDV isolates that has produced the best evidence for the involvement of carrier cattle in further infection of susceptible cattle.

In April, 1989 there was an isolated outbreak of FMD due to a type S.A.T. 2 strain of FMDV at Delken Farm, Mutorashanga, in the non-vaccinating zone of Zimbabwe (see Fig. 1). A sample isolate from this outbreak (Zim 8/89) was sequenced and found to be closely related to the virus responsible for an outbreak of FMD at Blackwaters Ranch, south of Harare, in 1987 (Zim 1/87). Movement records showed that cattle had been moved from Fountains Farm, a near neighbour of Blackwaters Ranch, to a market in February, 1987. These cattle were subsequently re-sold and moved to Delken Farm. FMD was not declared on Blackwaters Ranch until March, 1987, but the possibility remains that the cattle moved from Fountains Farm became FMDV carriers before their movement for sale and were responsible for the outbreak of FMD at Delken Farm in 1989.

Stronger circumstantial evidence for the role of FMDV carrier cattle in the epidemiology of FMD was gained from the analysis of field isolates collected from another isolated outbreak in the non-vaccinating zone of Zimbabwe in October, 1991 at Whaddon Chase Farm, Mvurwi (see Fig. 1). The sequence data from the S.A.T. 2 FMD viruses isolated from this outbreak were very similar to that of the isolates collected from a previous outbreak of FMD in 1989 near Gweru, south of Harare. Examination of movement records showed that cattle had moved to Whaddon Chase Farm immediately before the the FMD outbreak in 1991, via cattle sales. These animals had originated from Aberfoyle Farm, a holding not involved in the 1989 FMD outbreak at Gweru, but close enough for the cattle to have been vaccinated during the containment campaign.

Zimbabwean veterinary personnel revisited Aberfoyle Farm in 1991 and discovered the existence of cattle persistently infected with a strain of FMDV S.A.T. 2. The sequences of these isolates were very closely related to both the 1989 Gweru outbreak isolates and the 1991 Aberfoyle Farm isolates. This evidence is consistent with the theory that vaccinated cattle became persistently infected with FMDV, and subsequently transmitted the largely unchanged virus to susceptible cattle 18 months later following transportation, thereby establishing a further outbreak of FMD.

The apparent genomic stability of the carrier viruses isolated from cattle at Aberfoyle Farm over a 3 year period is supported by recent antigenicity studies on FMDV carrier isolates from cattle maintained at the Institute for Animal Health, Pirbright (J.Salt, unpublished data). Table 2 shows the reactivity of carrier isolates of type O FMDV against a panel of monoclonal antibodies. There was no major change in viral antigenicity over a period of 10 months.

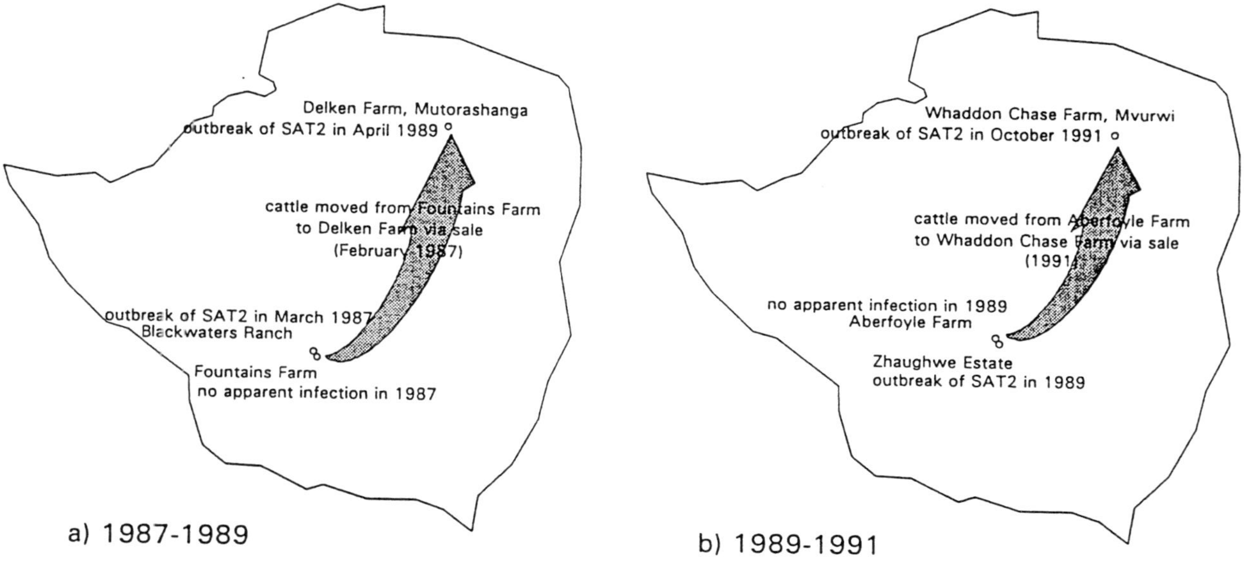

Figure 1. Suggested involvement of FMDV carrier cattle in outbreaks of FMD in Zimbabwe (N.J.Knowles).

Table 2. Reactivity of a panel of monoclonal antibodies with FMDV isolates from a long-term carrier cow. Values represent % recativity with homologous virus.

		Monoclonal antibody						
P-i[a]	Passage	B2	C6	C8	C9	D9	A8	G5
O_1 Saudi 8/88[b]		55	0	72	11	97	20	0
RV20								
5	BTY 1[c]	47	1	64	9	81	61	1
8	RS 1[d]	64	0	68	33	97	64	3
9	BTY 1	72	0	73	23	81	63	0
11	BTY 2[e]	34	0	44	17	72	84	2
12	BTY 1	56	0	61	17	91	49	1
15	BTY 2	49	4	69	11	82	74	1
17	BTY 2	33	0	50	7	55	90	1
18	BTY 2	60	1	66	11	74	60	0
18	RS 1	62	0	67	15	93	89	8
19	BTY 2	32	0	56	16	72	41	0
20	BTY 2	46	1	62	12	75	75	1
21	BTY 1	33	0	49	0	59	77	4
25	BTY 1	60	2	71	7	82	79	0
28	BTY 1	46	1	73	9	84	73	0
29	BTY 2	48	0	88	18	78	51	0
30	RS 1	69	0	73	15	85	77	7
33	BTY 2	66	1	79	8	79	64	2

[a]P-i, days post-infection.
[b]Original isolate used for cattle challenge.
[c]BTY 1, virus samples were the original isolations on BTY cells.
[d]RS 1, virus samples were passaged once in IB-RS-2 cells from the original BTY isolation.
[e]BTY 2, virus samples were passaged once in BTY cells from the original BTY isolation.

THE CARRIER THREAT

The successful transmission of FMDV from a carrier animal to a susceptible animal may be a rare event and occur under a particular set of circumstances for each of the participants. However, for any FMD-free region of the world the contact of susceptible livestock with FMDV carrier animals is an unacceptable concept. International trade in livestock and livestock products between FMD-free countries and countries in which FMD is endemic is rightly severely restricted. Quarantine, laboratory testing and guarantees of non-vaccinated status may be preconditions imposed on the entry of livestock from such countries. Following the decision of the Commission of E.C. to adopt a 'stamping out', non-vaccination policy for the control of FMD from 1992, prophlactic vaccination has ceased and the European herd is becoming increasingly more susceptible to FMDV.

The most significant threat represented by FMDV carrier animals is the introduction of FMDV into FMD-free regions, and to a lesser extent the potential introduction of new strains of FMDV into regions which are not FMD-free. There are two potential sources of FMDV carrier animals for a FMD-free region: external and internal. FMDV carriers may enter a country by the legal importation of animals wrongly certificated or identified, or the illegal entry of animals as a result of smuggling across international boundaries. The latter occurrence is encouraged as a result of the likely price differential existing between countries free from FMD and endemic countries because of the former's access to export markets.

Secondly, carrier animals may result from outbreaks of FMD within FMD-free countries if adherence to the 'stamping out' policy is inadequate to control an outbreak and a 'ring-vaccination' policy is resorted to for containment of the outbreak. In this situation many protected animals could be exposed to FMDV around an infection focus, and would necessarily have to be treated as potential FMDV carriers. The prolonged duration of persistent FMDV infection in cattle would require these animals to be monitored for at least 2.5 years. Obviously there is a risk that these cattle could become mixed with the susceptible population. In addition, challenge of susceptible cattle with low doses of FMDV, as may occur around a future outbreak on the edges of a virus plume, favours sub-clinical infection (Sutmoller et al, 1968) and therefore the possible production of undetected carriers that would have free movement around the country.

THE DIAGNOSIS OF PERSISTENT FMDV INFECTION

Current situation

The only available system for the identification of FMDV carriers is virus isolation in tissue culture and subsequent characterisation by ELISA. FMDV isolation on primary bovine thyroid cells (Snowdon, 1966) has been shown to be the most sensitive assay for the detection of FMDV, with equivalent sensitivity to cattle tongue inoculation (House and House, 1989). Whilst this system is adequate for the detection of FMDV in clinical samples collected during the acute stage of FMD, the low virus titre, the intermittent nature of virus recovery and the possible presence of neutralising antibody in probang samples from carrier animals may reduce the efficiency of virus detection.

Standard serological assays are not useful for the detection of persistent FMDV infection.

Serum antibody titres to structural proteins of FMDV are not significantly different in convalescent cattle that eliminate FMDV and those that remain persistently infected. Similarly vaccinated, protected cattle that become FMDV carriers post-challenge are serologically indistinguishable from non-carriers using conventional assays. Serology is further complicated by the occasional occurrence of carrier animals with no measurable serum antibody or titres that would be considered negative for the purposes of international trade (Hedger, 1968).

Future prospects

In view of the inadequacies of currently available techniques for the accurate identification of FMDV carriers, several approaches are being made to improve the situation. Bergmann et al (1993) recently suggested that the serological response to the non-structural proteins of FMDV was significantly prolonged in persistently infected cattle. The immunoblotting system used in this work is relatively cumbersome for routine diagnostic purposes. Several laboratories, including the European Community Reference Laboratory at Pirbright, are currently optimising ELISA techniques using cloned and expressed recombinant FMDV non-structural proteins for serological diagnostic purposes to replace the less sensitive gel immunodiffusion test previously employed for the detection of serum antibody to one of the non-structural proteins of FMDV, 3D or VIAA.

Isotype-specific ELISA analysis of secretory samples from FMD convalescent cattle has shown that there is a statistically significant difference in FMDV-specific IgA between carrier and non-carrier cattle (J S Salt, unpublished data). This relationship has been shown in probang fluid samples and saliva, which is a more readily obtainable sample for analysis (see Fig. 2). The prolonged secretion of FMDV-specific IgA in the fluids bathing the upper respiratory tract offers a potential means of FMDV carrier identification.

Molecular biological developments in the diagnosis of FMDV have recently been described which offer the potential for improved detection of a low genome copy number in clinical samples. House and Meyer (1993) and Amaral-Doel et al (1993) have developed assays utilising the polymerase chain reaction (PCR) for the detection of FMDV in probang fluid samples either directly or following inoculation of tissue culture. The exquisite sensitivity and potential for cross-serotype reactivity of these systems could be a major improvement in the diagnosis of FMDV carriers. However, the interpretation of a positive result by the direct assay still has to be determined in relation to the presence of replicating virus.

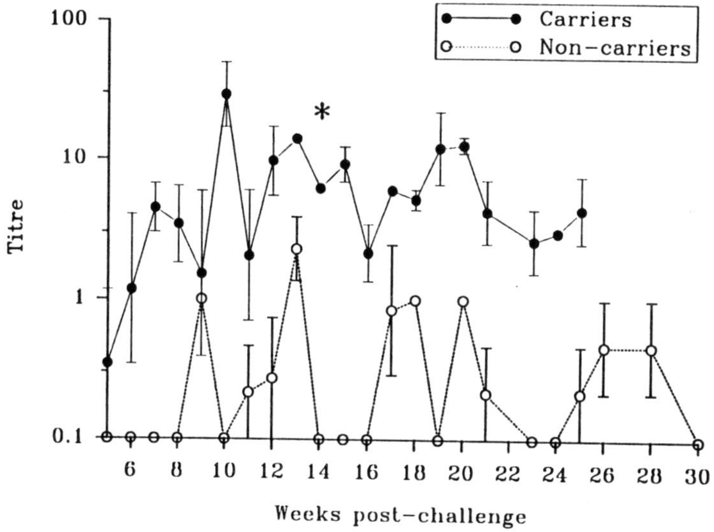

Figure 2. Type O FMDV-specific IgA titres in probang samples from FMDV carrier (n=4) and non-carrier (n=3) cattle. Points represent mean+/- S.E. * Marks the point beyond which the difference between the groups became significant ($p<0.01$)

CONCLUSION

There is accumulating evidence that animals persistently infected with FMDV are responsible for the establishment of further outbreaks of disease amongst susceptible livestock. Recent developments in rapid nucleotide sequencing have determined the stability of isolates collected from persistently infected cattle in Zimbabwe over periods of up to 3 years. Changes to E.C. policy for the control of FMD have resulted in the increasing susceptibility of the European herd. Therefore, enhanced awareness of the risks of importation or movement of FMDV carrier animals within the E.C. is required. To this end improved techniques for the detection of persistent infection with FMDV are anticipated, which can be used in more stringent control systems prior to importation. Further work is required to understand the *stress factors* that may be involved in the transmission of FMDV from carriers in an attempt to avoid further outbreaks of FMD initiated by FMDV carriers.

REFERENCES

Amaral-Doel, C.M.F., Owen, N.E., Ferris, N.P., Kitching, R.P. and Doel, T.R. (1993). Detection of foot-and-mouth disease viral sequences in clinical specimens and ethyleneimine-inactivated preparations by the polymerase chain reaction. Vaccine 11, 415-421.

Anderson, E.C., Doughty, W.J. and Anderson, J. (1974). The effect of repeated vaccination in an enzootic foot and mouth disease area on the incidence of virus carrier cattle. J. Hyg., Camb. 73, 229-235.

Anderson, E.C., Doughty, W.J. and Anderson, J. (1976). The role of sheep and goats in the epizootiology of foot and mouth disease in Kenya. J. Hyg. 76, 395-402.

Anderson, E.C., Foggin, C., Atkinson, M., Sorenson, K.J., Madekurozva, R.L. and Nqindi, J. (1993). The role of wild animals, other than buffalo, in the current epidemiology of foot-and-mouth disease in Zimbabwe. Epidemiol. Infect. 111, 559-563.

Auge de Mello, P., Honigman, M.H., Fernandez, M.V. and Gomes, I. (1966). Further information on the survival of modified foot and mouth disease virus in cattle. Bull. Off. int. Epiz. 73, 489-505.

Bengis, R.G., Thomson, G.R., Hedger, R.S., de Vos, V. and Pini, A. (1986). Foot and mouth disease and the African buffalo (Syncerus caffer). Onderstepoort J. Vet. Res. 53, 69-73.

Bergmann, I.E., de Mello, P.A., Neitzert, E., Beck, E. and Gomes, I. (1993). Diagnosis of persistent aphthovirus infection and its differentiation from vaccination response in cattle by use of enzyme-linked immunoelectrotransfer blot analysis with bioengineered nonstructural viral antigens. Am. J. Vet. Res. 54, 825-831.

Burrows, R. (1966). Studies on the carrier state of cattle exposed to foot and mouth disease virus. J. Hyg., Camb. 64, 81-90.

Burrows, R. (1968). The persistence of FMDV in sheep. J. Hyg., Camb. 66, 633-640.

Burrows, R., Mann, J.A., Greig, A., Chapman, W.G. and Goodridge, D. (1971). The growth and persistence of foot-and-mouth disease virus in the bovine mammary gland. J. Hyg., Camb. 69, 307-321.

Condy, J.B., Hedger, R.S., Hamblin, C. and Barnett, I.T.R. (1985). The duration of the foot and mouth disease virus carrier state in African buffalo. Comp. Immun. Microbiol. Infect. Dis. 8, 259-265.

Cottral, G.E. (1969). Persistence of foot and mouth disease virus in animals, their products and the environment. Bull. Off. int. Epiz. 71, 549-568.

Diez, J., Hofner, M., Domingo, E. and Donaldson, A.I. (1990). Foot and mouth disease virus strains isolated from persistently infected cell cultures are attenuated for mice and cattle. Virus Research 18, 3-8.

Donaldson, A.I. (1987). Foot and mouth disease: the principal features. Irish Vet. J. 41, 325-327.

Donaldson, A.I., Gibson, C.F., Oliver, R., Hamblin, C. and Kitching, R.P. (1987). Infection of cattle by airborne foot-and-mouth disease virus: minimal doses with O_1 and S.A.T. 2 strains. Res. Vet. Sci. 43, 339-346.

Donaldson, A.I. and Kitching, R.P. (1989). Transmission of foot and mouth disease by vaccinated cattle following natural challenge. Rev. Vet. Sci. 46, 9-14.

Hedger, R.S. (1968). The isolation and characterisation of foot-and-mouth disease virus from clinically normal herds of cattle in Botswana. J. Hyg., Camb. 66, 27-36.

Hedger, R.S. (1970). Observations on the carrier state and related antibody titres during an outbreak of foot and mouth disease. J. Hyg., Camb. 68, 53-60.

Hedger, R.S. and Stubbins, A.G.J. (1971). The carrier state in foot and mouth disease, and the probang test. State Vet. J. 26, 45-50.

Hedger, R.S. and Condy, J.B. (1985). Transmission of foot and mouth disease from African buffalo virus carriers to bovines. Vet. Record 117, 205.

House, C. and House, J.A. (1989). Evaluation of techniques to demonstrate foot-and-mouth disease virus in bovine tongue epithelium: comparison of the sensitivity of cattle, mice, primary cell cultures, cryopreserved cell cultures and established cell lines. Vet. Microbiol. 20, 99-109.

House, C. and Meyer, R.F. (1993). The detection of foot-and-mouth disease virus in oesophageal-pharyngeal samples by a polymerase chain reaction technique. J. Virol. Methods 43, 1-6.

Kaaden, O., Eissner, G. and Bohm, H.O. (1975). Studies on permanent virus excretors in cattle vaccinated and experimentally infected with foot and mouth disease. Anim. Res. Dev. 1, 20-33.

Loeffler, F. and Frosch, P. (1898). Berichte der Kommission zur Erforschung der Maul-und-Klauenseuche bei dem Institut fur Infektionskrankheiten in Berlin. Zentrablatt fur Bakteriologie, Parasitenkunde, Infectionskrankheiten und Hygiene, Abteilungen I, Original 23, 371-391.

Mohler, J.R. (1926). Foot and mouth disease with special reference to the outbreaks in California, 1924 and Texas, 1924 and 1926. U.S. Dept. of Agric. Circ. 400, 1-82.

Pay, T.W.F. (1988). FMD in sheep and goats - a review. FMD Bulletin 26, 2-13.

Rossi, M.S., Sadir, A.M., Schudel, A.A. and Palma, G.L. (1988). The detection of foot and mouth disease virus with DNA probes in bovine oesophageal-pharyngeal fluids. Arch. Virol. 99, 67-74.

Snowdon, W.A. (1966). Growth of foot-and-mouth disease virus in monolayer cultures of calf thyroid cells. Nature 210, 1079-1080.

Sutmoller, P. and Gaggero, A. (1965). Foot and mouth disease carriers. Vet. Record 77, 968-969.

Sutmoller, P., McVicar, J.W. and Cottral, G.E. (1968). The epizootiological importance of foot-and-mouth disease carriers. Arch. fur ges. Virusforsch. 23, 227-235.

van Bekkum, J.G., Frenkel, H.S.,Frederiks, H.H.J. and Frenkel, S. (1959). Observations on the carrier state of cattle exposed to foot and mouth disease virus. Tijdschr. Diergeneesk. 84, 1159-1164.

van Bekkum, J.G., Straver, P.J., Bool, P.H. and Frenkel, S. (1966). Further information on the persistence of infective foot-and-mouth disease virus in cattle exposed to virulent virus strains. Bull. Off. int. Epiz. 65, 1949-1965.

van Bekkum, J.G. (1973). The carrier state in foot and mouth disease. In: Pollard M. (Ed.), Proc. 2nd. Int. Conf. on FMD.; Gustav Stern Foundation Inc., New York; pp. 45-50.

Waldmann, O., Trautwein, K. and Pyl, G. (1931). Persistence of foot and mouth disease virus in the body and secretions of recovered animals. Zentbl. Bakt. Parasit. Infect. Abt. 1 Orig. 121, 19.

AN EPIDEMIOLOGICAL INVESTIGATION OF DISEASES OF FARMED ATLANTIC SALMON - PRELIMINARY FINDINGS

S.B. WHEATLEY*, E.A. GOODALL*, F.D. MENZIES** and M. F. McLOUGHLIN**

A computerised database of epidemiological data relating to the marine phase of Atlantic salmon culture in Ireland has been established by the Veterinary Science Department at The Queen's University of Belfast. The establishment of this database is considered essential for the development of effective control strategies by the salmon farming industry following outbreaks of disease, particularly with respect to Pancreas Disease (PD). This paper presents the preliminary findings from interrogation of the database.

PANCREAS DISEASE

Pancreas Disease is regarded as a serious threat to the economic production of farmed Atlantic salmon in Ireland (Branson, 1988). It is estimated that PD cost the Irish salmon farming industry in the region of 5 to 6 million pounds in 1987 (Branson, 1988). This estimated loss was based on a mean mortality level of 10% per farm in 1987. The average mortality reported due to PD in 1990 was 25% (Wheatley, 1992).

PD affects farmed Atlantic salmon during their marine stage of growth, normally in their first year at sea. PD was initially described in Scotland in 1976 (Munro *et al.*, 1984). The condition is now thought to occur in all of the major salmon farming countries of Europe and also in the USA (Kent & Elston, 1987; Poppe *et al.*, 1989).

Clinical signs of PD are a sudden decrease in feeding response, listlessness, a tendency to group in cage corners close to the water surface and the production of white faecal casts. Severely affected fish do not feed, rapidly lose weight and a proportion of fish never recover. This gives rise to the variability in size which in turn leads to considerable management problems. Affected fish show increased susceptibility to other diseases and fish farmers have the added problem that it is not possible to use oral treatment for those secondary conditions.

In Ireland, a condition associated with PD termed Sudden Death Syndrome (SDS), has been described (Rodger *et al.*, 1991). Deaths from SDS occur six to eight weeks after the diagnosis of PD. It has been proposed by Rodger *et al.* (1991) that SDS occurs due to nutritional deficiency and exertion following the pancreatic lesions associated with PD.

* Biometrics Department, The Queen's University of Belfast, Newforge Lane, Belfast BT9 5PX
** Veterinary Sciences Division, Department of Agriculture NI, Stormont, Belfast BT4 3SD

There is considerable evidence to support a viral aetiology for PD, although an infectious agent has not yet been isolated or identified (Raynard *et al.*, 1992). Consequently it has been difficult to devise control measures for dealing with PD (Raynard *et al.* 1992).

The main aims of this project are firstly to establish a database of production, disease, environment and management data from Irish marine salmon farms and secondly to analyse these data to identify critical factors, trends or patterns preceding and during disease outbreaks. This approach may assist in identifying the risk factors associated with disease and devising practical control measures for diseases such as PD.

MATERIALS AND METHODS

The methods used for identifying farms for intensive monitoring and the data collection methods used have been previously described by Menzies *et al.* (1992).

Salmon farm database

Data were standardised in relation to each site and each cage within a site, and the variables were further categorised as constant, categorical or continuous variables (Tab. 1). Continuous variables were computed as an average over fortnightly intervals. Categorical data also refer to events within the same two week interval.

Table. 1. Examples of the types of variable recorded on the salmon farm database.

Variable type	Variable
Constant site data	Year farming started at this site Water depth at mean low spring tide Single or multiple generation site Length of fallowing before smolt input
Continuous site data	Water temperature Dissolved oxygen Salinity Chlorophyll
Categorical site data	Occurrence of any of the major diseases Laboratory confirmation of diagnosis
Constant cage data	Cage type Depth and volume of cage Single or block of cages Vaccination Average weight and number at transfer Transfer method Feeding method
Continuous cage data	Number and percentage mortalities
Categorical cage data	Feed manufacturer Feed type and size Inclusion of pigment

Figure 1 illustrates the relationship between the different files held within the database.

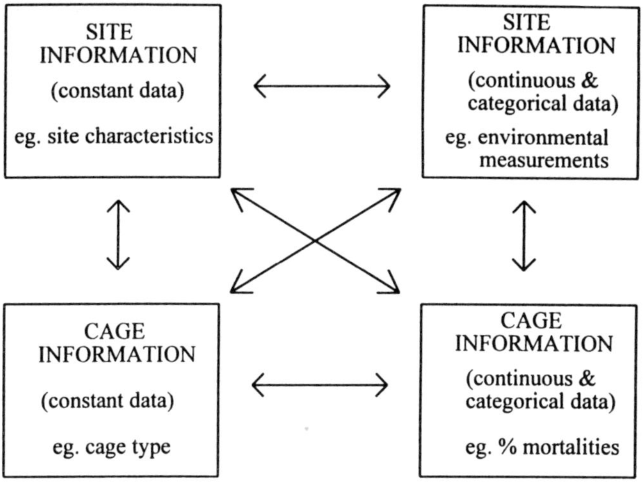

Figure 1. Diagramatic representation of the relationship between files within the salmon farm database.

The database system was configured using the software package ORACLE, a relational database management system available on a VAX 6320 supermini computer which has 64 megabytes of main memory and 7 gigabytes of disk backing storage. The use of ORACLE enables the formation of extract files of categorised subsets of data before subsequent analysis by other software packages.

Statistical analysis

The interval between smolt input and December inclusively during the first year at sea was studied. This avoided the complications of grading and transfer of stocks which occur on farm following the first winter at sea. Percentage mortality within each two weekly interval was used as an indicator of production. Biomass would be a more appropriate measure of production, however estimations of the average weight of salmon within each cage were infrequent so that biomass in individual cages could not be accurately assessed on any of the sites.

Routine statistical analyses, such as the Gossets t-test, analysis of variance and multiple regression analysis were carried out using SPSS. A suite of specially developed FORTRAN programs were used for time series analysis of the data. This software provides comprehensive facilities for computing moving averages and allows for linear combinations of variables to be correlated over any selected time period with mortality data at coincident or lagged time periods.

RESULTS

The database currently contains information on 13 million fish from eleven sites over a five year period.

Mortality rates due to the significant diseases of farmed Atlantic salmon in Ireland

Initial information from a questionnaire survey conducted in 1990 indicated that the most significant disease conditions were PD, SDS, vibriosis and furunculosis and sea lice infestation (Menzies *et al.*, 1992).

The mortality rates associated with the major diseases of the Irish salmon farming industry from 1988 to 1992 have been quantified using the salmon farm database (Tab. 2).

Table 2. Overall mortality rates associated with outbreaks of the major disease conditions on farms recorded on the database.

Disease	% of total mortality	% of smolt input
PD and SDS[a]	51.3	14.1
Vibriosis[b]	10.8	3.0
Furunculosis	2.6	0.7
Miscellaneous (eg. transport losses, storm damage)	35.3	9.6

Note: a Where concurrent outbreaks of vibriosis or furunculosis occurred, mortalities during this period were excluded from the calculation of PD and SDS mortality.

b Where concurrent outbreaks of furunculosis occurred, mortalities during this period were excluded from the calculation of vibriosis mortality. Mortalities occurring during outbreaks of vibriosis in association with PD or SDS were included here.

The overall mortality from smolt input to sea until the end of December of the first year was 27.41%. Half of the overall mortalities were associated with PD/SDS. This estimate of PD associated mortality may be conservative, because in any period where concurrent outbreaks of vibriosis or furunculosis occurred, losses were attributed to these latter conditions alone. Mortality levels which were attributable to other causes, for example, transport losses, storm damage and algal blooms cumulated to 35.3% of overall mortality.

Time series analysis of mortality curves during PD outbreaks

Time series analysis of mortality data was used to determine if patterns of mortality during an outbreak of PD indicated that the disease is primarily caused by an infectious agent. The hypothesis that successive peaks in mortality between cages were not dependent on each other, that is, that mortality events in neighbouring cages bear no relation to each other, was tested. The mortality data from a group of cages (moored adjacent to one another) on one site

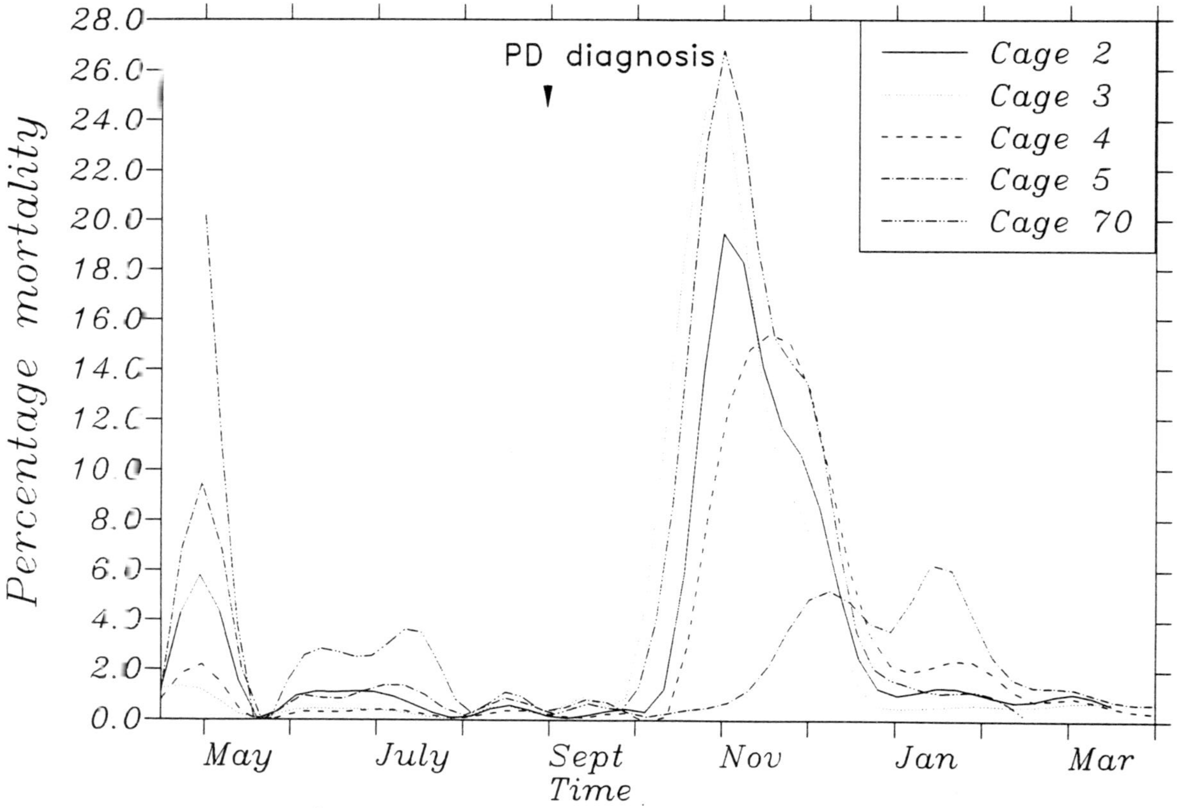

Figure 2: Fortnightly percentage mortality from input 1990 in each cage at a site suffering PD in August 1990.

were used as an example of this analysis (Fig. 2). In 1990, transport losses were high (April-May). Mortality during June and July was attributed to outbreaks of a condition known as Summer Lesion Syndrome. PD was first noticed on this site on 28 August .

Adjacent cages were paired and regression analysis was carried out on each paired set of data. Regression analysis was carried out on mortality figures which had been time-lagged against each other to determine if mortality patterns were synchronous. A straight line was obtained for cage pairs 3 and 70, 70 and 2 and 2 and 4 when the time lag was zero ($p<0.001$). Cages 4 and 5 showed a straight line relationship when the mortality figures were lagged by four weeks against one another ($p<0.10$). PD did occur in cage 5, but this cage showed a slower increase in mortality and lower overall mortality levels. Time series analysis of mortality data from another site where cages were moored approximately 30 metres apart showed a consistent time lag of four weeks ($P<0.05$).

The proportion of cases in which the first cage or group of cages diagnosed with PD was the most severely affected by the disease is shown in Tab. 3. In this analysis, a cage group is defined as an aggregate of cages which are moored at equal distances from one another. The distance between cage groups must be at least twice the distance that occurs between neighbouring cages within a group. In half of the outbreaks it was the first group of fish suffering PD which showed the highest mortality in an outbreak.

Table 3. The percentage of outbreaks of PD in which the first cage or group of cages suffering PD had the highest level of mortality in the outbreak.

	Within cage groups	Between cage groups
Total number of outbreaks	40	14
First cage/group of cages suffering PD had the highest level of mortality	52.5	50.0
First cage/group of cages suffering PD did not have the highest level of mortality	22.5	36.0
Mortality patterns were inconclusive due to concurrent disease conditions	7.5	7.0
Insufficient mortality data	17.5	7.0

<u>The effect of site management methods on total mortality levels</u>

The total mortality data for each year from each site were classified as either:

1. Fallowed or unfallowed.
2. Single generation or multiple generation.
3. Sites where harvested fish were bled on site or sites where harvested fish were not bled on site.

In this analysis, sites were classed as fallowed if all stocks were removed from the site for a period of at least 3 weeks prior to the input of smolts.

When a site is fallowed it is normally stocked with a single year-class in the following year. However, in three cases the sites were stocked with one year-class only, but fallowing was not practiced. Similarly, if a site contains a single generation only, it is less likely that fish will be harvested on site. In general then these three site management practices are related and are used in conjunction with one another.

Analysis showed that sites where fallowing, use of single generation stock and harvesting off site were practiced had significantly lower total mortality levels (Tab. 4).

Table 4. The effect of site management methods on total site mortality: fallowing, single generation sites and bleeding of harvested fish on site.

Variable	n	Mean	SE	t	Significance
Fallowed	9	19.6	3.23	2.26	0.033
Not fallowed	25	30.1	3.36		
Single generation	12	20.0	3.52	2.29	0.030
Multiple generation	22	31.3	3.49		
Fish not bled on site	15	21.0	3.28	2.26	0.031
Fish bled on site	19	32.3	3.80		

<u>The effect of single generation rearing on the mean number of sea lice treatments applied per cage annually at each site</u>

Fourteen years of data detailing the number of Dichlorvos treatments for sea lice administered to each cage on site in the first year at sea were available. These were classed as either single or multiple generation sites (Tab. 5).

Table 5. The effect of using single generation sites on the mean number of lice treatments required per cage annually. Results of a t-test carried out on all available data, which includes sites using Dichlorvos only (a), and of a t-test carried out on data excluding those sites using Dichlorvos only (b).

Variable	n	Mean	SE	t	Significance
Single generation	4	1.6	0.63	2.76[a]	0.017
Multiple generation	10	4.8	0.95		
Single generation	3	1.4	0.83	0.89[b]	0.415
Multiple generation	4	2.4	0.77		

The mean number of sea lice treatments with Dichlorvos in both groups is quite low. This is because in both groups, a variety of control measures were applied in conjunction with Dichlorvos, reducing the overall need for Dichlorvos treatment.

The results of this analysis show that the mean number of Dichlorvos treatments required was significantly lower in the groups practising single generation rearing.

In seven of the years tested here, Dichlorvos was the only method used for sea lice treatment. There was one such year in the single generation group and six in the multiple generation group. To remove the effect of Dichlorvos only treated sites, these sites were excluded and the t-values recomputed, the result of this analysis was not significant.

DISCUSSION

This project has facilitated the collection and analysis of the most accurate disease and production information which is available from the Irish salmon industry. Comparisons can now be made between the eleven sites which are distributed throughout Ireland with respect to the four different types of parameter namely, production, management, disease and environment.

The mortality rates associated with PD demonstrated unequivocally the severity of this condition in Ireland from 1988 to 1992. PD resulted in 14.1% mortality of total smolt input in the first year at sea. Setbacks in growth and consequent runting as a result of PD must be included in any assessment of the economic impact of this condition. Furthermore, the high mortality levels associated with PD usually occur from late summer onwards, when the stock have grown considerably and hence are more valuable.

It is evident from this study that PD and SDS cause considerable losses on Irish sea farms. Control measures for this condition are crucial for the future of this industry.

There has been controversy in the literature over the definition and outcome of PD in farmed salmon. In general, outbreaks of PD in Scotland result in low mortality levels, ranging from 1-5% (Munro *et al.* , 1984; Ferguson *et al.*, 1986; McVicar, 1986; McVicar, 1987). American, Norwegian, French and Spanish research all indicate that mortality levels due to PD can be high but variable (Kent & Elston, 1987; Poppe *et al.*, 1989; Barja, 1992; Baudin-Laurencin, 1992). This is consistent with the findings of PD mortality in Ireland revealed by this study.

It is possible that these contradictory reports of mortality levels associated with PD may be because of different manifestations of this disease in different salmon producing areas. However, the variability in PD associated mortality could be related to the fact that Scottish workers generally attribute mortality during PD to what they describe as secondary conditions, such as furunculosis, vibriosis, sea lice infestation and failure to feed (McVicar, 1987). In this study any mortality associated with vibriosis or furunculosis outbreaks was excluded from the calculation of PD associated mortality levels. Exclusion of these mortalities had little effect on the severe mortality levels attributable to PD. It was not possible to attribute mortality to either sea lice infestation or failure to feed. Therefore the impact of these conditions on mortality during PD remains unknown.

The analysis of mortality data from neighbouring cages indicated that the mortality patterns were similar during PD outbreaks in all cases tested and that the pattern was consistent with that expected for an infectious fish disease (Austin & Austin, 1989). Sites in which cages were located further apart showed a slower progression of PD through the cages. This is consistent with the current view that PD is likely to be an infectious disease (Raynard *et al.*, 1992). The finding that the first cage in a group of cages to suffer PD is often the worst affected is less easily explained.

The following hypotheses may be responsible for the observed mortality pattern:

(a) The first cage to suffer PD had a higher susceptibility due to the presence of a predisposing factor(s) as yet unidentified.
(b) Management techniques implemented once PD was identified allowed for some control over the severity of the outbreak.
(c) Cages which suffer mortalities later in a PD outbreak may have developed a degree of immunity to the infectious agent which is thought to cause PD.

Further analysis of the information that has been collected since the project began may identify the predisposing factors associated with PD outbreaks.

PD should be treated as an infectious disease on the farm Control measures should include restricting movement of infected fish stocks, disinfection of personnel and equipment and the application of fallowing and single year class sites. These practical measures should reduce the impact of PD/SDS on the farm.

In general, the practice of fallowing, single generation rearing and of harvesting away from other generations of fish have beneficial effects overall on Irish sea farms. Bron, *et al.* (1993) showed that the numbers of *Lepeophtheirus salmonis* (an ectoparasite of salmon) were reduced for several months post fallowing, with much less need for the use of chemotherapy. Fallowing can also reduce the occurrence of other infectious diseases of Atlantic salmon culture. In addition, fallowing prevents the enrichment which can occur due to intensive culture in inshore waters (O'Connor, *et al.*, 1993). Enrichment of the mariculture environment can have deleterious effects on fish health (Gowan & McLusky, 1988).

By practising single generation rearing the potential for horizontal transmission of pathogenic organisms between age groups of differing susceptibilities is reduced. This is apparent in the data on the mean number of sea lice treatments and number of year-classes per site. This analysis revealed that there were fewer Dichlorvos treatments applied at the single generation sites, but this result was not statistically significant. The limited data currently available probably reduced the significance of this result. It is interesting that the one case in which a single generation site used only Dichlorvos for sea lice control, had a very low mean number of sea lice treatments.

Finally, the analysis has shown that harvesting of growers on site where relatively newly introduced fish are reared has a deleterious effect on fish health. Harvesting should take place away from other growing populations of fish.

CONCLUSIONS

Further work using the database will allow quantification of the multifactoral aspects of PD and the other economically important diseases of farmed Atlantic salmon in Ireland. The salmon farm database will be of invaluable benefit to the Irish salmon industry in quantifying health problems and devising effective control measures for profitable production of farmed Atlantic Salmon in Ireland.

These preliminary findings show that if measures such as fallowing and single generation rearing are carried out on Irish sea farms, mortality levels are reduced. These site management methods also significantly reduce the number of sea lice treatments, possibly indicating a reduction in ectoparasite infestation levels. This can only be beneficial to the overall fish health, production and environmental impact of intensive mariculture sites in Ireland.

ACKNOWLEDGEMENTS

We wish to thank the Irish Salmon Growers Association and An Bord Iascaigh Mhara. The assistance of farmers, veterinary laboratories and environmental monitoring firms are gratefully acknowledged.

REFERENCES

Austin, B. and Austin, D.A. (1989). Methods for the microbiological examination of fish and shellfish. Ellis Horwood Ltd , Chicester.

Barja, J. (1992). Pancreas disease in Galicia. In: Pancreas disease of Atlantic salmon. Proceedings of a European commission workshop. R. Raynard, G. Houghton and A.L.S. Munro (Eds.) Scottish Office Aquaculture Report. No 1, p4.

Baudin-Laurencin, F. (1992). Pancreas disease in France. In: Pancreas disease of Atlantic salmon. Proceedings of a European commission workship. R. Raynard, G. Houghton and A.L.S. Munro (Eds.) Scottish Office Aquaculture Report. No 1, p4.

Branson, E.J. (1988). Review of Pancreas disease. Unpublished report produced by Stirling University, May 1988, p12.

Bron, J.E., Sommerville, C., Wotten, R. and Rae, G.H. (1993). Fallowing of marine Atlantic salmon, *Salmo salar* L., farms as a method for control fo the sea lice, *Lepeophtheirus salmonis* (Kroyer, 1837). J. Fish. Dis. **16**: 487-493.

Ferguson, H.W., Roberts, R.J., Richards, R.H., Collins, R.O. and Rice, D.A. (1986). Severe degenerative cardiomyopathy associated with Pancreas disease in Atlantic salmon, *Salmo salar* L. J. Fish. Dis. **20**: 95-98.

Gowen, R.J. and McLusky, D.S. (1988). How farms affect their surroundings. Fish Farmer. Sept/Oct. 1988, 33-34.

Kent, M.L. and Elston, R.A. (1987). Pancreas disease in pen-reared Atlantic salmon in North America. Bull. Eur. Ass. Fish Pathol. **7** (2): 29-31.

O'Connor, B., Costelloe, J., Dinneen, P. and Faull, J. (1993). The effect of harrowing and fallowing on sediment quality under a salmon farm on the west coast of Ireland. International Council for the Exploration of the Sea. CM 1993/F:19. Mariculture Committee.

McVicar, A.H. (1986). Observations on pancreas disease of sea farmed Atlantic salmon (*Salmo salar* L.). International Council for the Exploration of the Sea. CM 1986/F:3. Mariculture Committee.

McVicar, A.H. (1987). Pancreas disease of farmed Atlantic salmon *Salmo salar*, in Scotland: epidemiology and early pathology. Aquaculture **67**: 71-78.

Menzies, F.D., Goodall, E.A., McLoughlin, M.F. and Wheatley, S.B. (1992). Computerised monitoring of disease and production in farmed Atlantic salmon (*Salmo salar*). Proceedings of a SVEPM Conference held in Edinburgh on 1-3 April 1992, p 138-147.

Munro, A.L.S., Ellis, A.E., McVicar, A.H., McLay, H.A. and Needham, E.A. (1984). An exocrine pancreas disease of farmed Atlantic salmon in Scotland. Holgolander Meeresuntersuchungen 37: 571-586.

Poppe, T., Rimstad, E. and Hyllseth, B. (1989). Pancreas disease in Atlantic salmon (*Salmo salar* L.) postsmolts infected with Infectious Pancreatic Necrosis Virus (IPNv). Bull. Eur. Ass. Fish Pathol. **9** (4) 83-85.

Raynard, R., Houghton, G. and Munro, A.L.S. (1992). Pancreas disease of Atlantic salmon: Proceedings of a European Commision workshop. Scottish Office Aquaculture Report No 1, p15.

Rodger, H.D., Murphy, T.M., Drinan, E.M. and Rice, D.A. (1991). Acute skeletal myopathy in farmed Atlantic salmon *Salmo salar*. Dis. aquat. Org. **12**: 17-23.

Wheatley, S.B. (1992). Salmon farming epidemiology project update. Aquaculture Ireland, Winter 1992, p 24-26.

CONTAGIOUS BOVINE PLEUROPNEUMONIA (CBPP) SURVEILLANCE IN SWITZERLAND: A PILOT STUDY

STÄRK, K.D.C.*, VICARI, A.† AND NICOLET, J.†

Contagious bovine pleuropneumonia (CBPP) is a highly contagious disease caused by *Mycoplasma (M.) mycoides subsp. mycoides* SC, affecting the lungs of adult cattle, domesticated buffaloes, bisons, yaks and zebus (Provost et al., 1987). The classical clinical signs are typical of acute pleuropneumonia, but chronic cases are also common and their detection is a major obstacle to disease control. Due to its economical impact, CBPP is included in the list 'A' diseases of the Office International des Epizooties (O.I.E.).

By the end of the 19th century CBPP was eradicated in Europe. But since 1980 outbreaks have occurred in France, Portugal, Spain and Italy (ter Laak, 1992). In Switzerland the last case to be confirmed dates back to 1895. Nevertheless in 1992, several Swiss cattle which had been exported to Italy were shown to be serologically positive for anti-CBPP antibodies. Consequently, this incident raised the question of the CBPP-disease free status of Switzerland, and the impact on trade. Based on a guideline worked out by an *ad hoc* expert group of the O.I.E. (1993), a pilot project was initiated in Switzerland with the objectives 1) to provide valid data on CBPP prevalence in the national cattle population, and 2) to make suggestions for a reliable surveillance system, including the discussion of practicability.

FREEDOM FROM DISEASE

In order to acquire disease-free status, the requirements of the O.I.E. must be met. Objective data will have to form the basis for such decisions. The O.I.E. has already published guidelines for the declaration of "freedom from disease" in the context of rinderpest (1989). These guidelines have been adapted to CBPP (O.I.E., 1993, Fig. 1) and can be considered to be of general applicability. The concept consists of a gradual declaration of three different stages of "freedom", which can be obtained when certain criteria and time limits have been met. An

* Inst. of Virology and Immunoprophylaxis, PO Box , CH-3147 Mittelhäusern
† Inst. for Veterinary Bacteriology, University of Berne, Länggassstrasse 122, CH-3012 Berne

essential part of this approach is a system of disease surveillance, which is necessary to provide epidemiologically sound evidence for the freedom from disease and thus forms the basis for its declaration by the O.I.E. Besides a reporting system for signs of disease by veterinary services and livestock owners, the O.I.E. requires an active surveillance adequate to detect clinical signs or other indications of the disease if they were present. Surveillance also implies, that action will follow from the discovery of evidence of disease or infection.

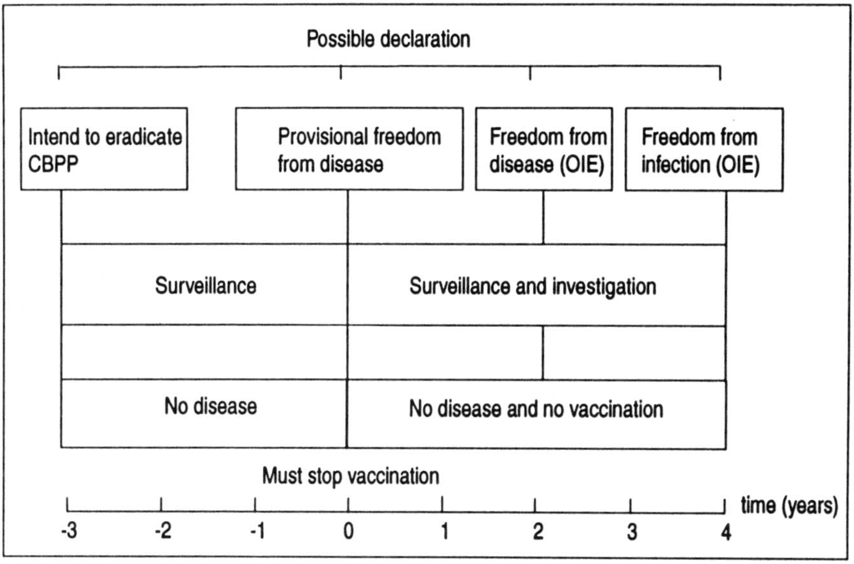

Fig. 1. Requirements for the declaration of "freedom from disease" and "freedom from infection" (O.I.E., 1993)

METHODS

Following the O.I.E. guidelines (1993), a system was developed in which the slaughterhouses are the primary sources of data.

Out of the more than 1'500 registered abattoirs 131 larger enterprises (>300 cattle killed in 1991) perform 87.8% of all slaughters in cattle (Table 1). The veterinarians in charge of meat inspection in these slaughterhouses were asked to participate in the study and 108 (82%) agreed to do so.

Table 1. Number and throughput of Swiss abattoirs (1991)

Abattoir size = #cattle slaughtered in 1991	#abattoirs	(# in study)	Total #cattle slaughtered in this group	Cumul. %
≥ 20'000	12	(12)	410'831	49.9
5'000 - 19'999	21	(17)	225'738	77.4
1'000 - 4'999	21	(17)	43'412	82.6
300 - 999	77	(62)	42'778	87.8
1 - 299	1'452	(0)	100'169	100
Total	1'583		822'928	

The meat inspectors were invited to a seminar, provided with illustrated information material, and instructed how to check, during routine meat inspection, the lungs of cattle older than 6 months for the specific lesions of CBPP. These lesions include distended interlobular septa and hepatisation ('Marble lung'), and sequestra containing necrotic material accompanied by hypertrophy of bronchial lymph nodes. These gross pathological signs are assumed to be pathognomonic for CBPP (Provost et al., 1987).

Suspect organs were sent to the Institute for Veterinary Bacteriology in Berne for microbiologic investigation, including complete bacteriological examination, the search for mycoplasmas following the protocols recommended by the O.I.E. (1992), as well as macroscopical and histological description of the lesions.

Additionally, a number of inconspicuous control lungs, along with lymph nodes and blood samples, had been collected in 7 abattoirs using systematic random sampling. These samples were examined bacteriologically as well as serologically, the latter using the standardized CF-test recommended by the O.I.E. (1992).

RESULTS

From June 1993 to November 1993, 84 suspect organs were turned in for examination. During this time period, the participating abattoirs performed approximately 200'000 slaughters of adult cattle (1 suspect lung on 2'600 inspected animals, <0.1%). The geographical distribution of the cattle with suspect lung lesions is shown in Fig. 2.

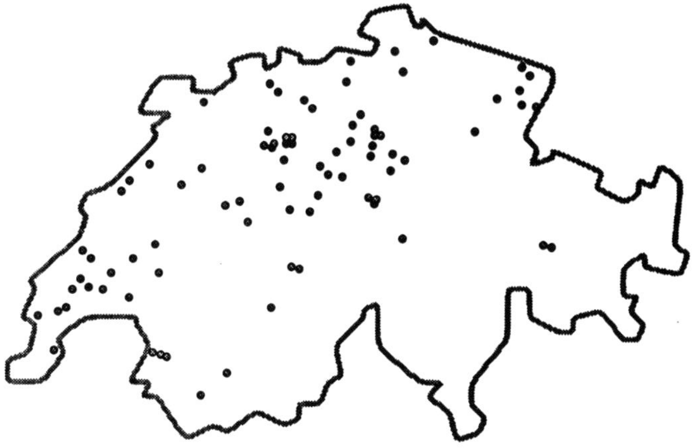

Fig. 2. Geographical distribution of cattle with suspect lung lesions

The results of the bacteriologic examinations are summarized in Table 2. The search for *M. mycoides subsp. mycoides* SC was negative in all lungs. The isolation of *Actinomyces pyogenes*, *Fusobacterium necrophorum* and/or mixed anaerobic flora was usually correlated with abscesses. Evidence for the presence of antibiotics could be found in 13 lungs, but these lungs showed neither macroscopically nor histologically typical lesions.

Table 2. Bacteriological diagnosis of suspected lungs

Bacteriological diagnosis	#isolations	(%)
Actinomyces pyogenes, *Fusobacterium necrophorum* and/or mixed anaerobic flora	43	(45.2)
Pasteurella haemolytica	6	(6.3)
Mycoplasma bovis	7	(7.4)
other Mycoplasma[a]	5	(5.3)
other bacteria	10	(10.5)
sterile or negative	24	(25.3)
Total	95[b]	

a. *Mycoplasma bovirhinis* (4), *Mycoplasma argini* (1)
b. more than one diagnosis in 11 cases

Out of the 72 control lungs, 6 were contaminated with *Streptococci viridans*, *E.coli* or mixed flora, the rest were sterile. Using the standardized CF-test recommended by the O.I.E., only one of 67 blood samples taken together with the control lungs reacted positively for anti-CBPP antibodies (titer 1/20++).

Despite the negative bacteriological results concerning *M. mycoides subsp. mycoides* SC, 6 pathologically particularly suspicious cases were traced back to the herds of origin, and blood samples taken for serological investigation from all adult cattle during a follow-up visit. The results are given in Table 3.

Table 3. Serological results of blood sampled on 6 farms

Farm ID	#reacting samples (total *#samples* taken)		titre
16	0	(19)	-
20	0	(23)	-
22	0	(9)	-
23	0	(37)	-
36	1	(21)	1/10+++
69	1	(15)	1/10++
Total	2	(124)	

DISCUSSION AND CONCLUSIONS

In order to be able to demonstrate that Switzerland is free from CBPP, the conduction of a surveillance system is essential. This programme should be designed such that it would have a very high probability of detecting the presence of disease. The outbreaks registered in Europe since 1980 showed a low morbidity and a very low mortality (ter Laak, 1992). Most of the cases were chronic, which is characteristic in an endemic situation. This pattern may be due to favourable climatic conditions and the use of anti-microbial or anti-inflammatory drugs that can mask the clinical signs. Therefore, clinical signs are not a reliable indicator for the disease. A further possibility to detect infected animals is systematic serological testing for anti-CBPP antibodies. However, the probably low prevalence of reactors as well as the possibility of non-specific reactions (Etheridge et al., 1976, Poumarat et al., 1989, Regalla et al., 1990) are prohibitive to any efficient large scale screening programme. There remains a CBPP surveillance system based on searching for the distinct gross pathological lesions of

CBPP during routine meat inspection procedures. In Switzerland, all slaughtered animals are subjected to meat inspection. This inspection includes palpation and section of the lungs and bronchial lymph nodes and is performed by veterinarians or trained laymen. Such a system should be a sensitive means to detect the disease and has therefore also been recommended by the O.I.E. (1993) as the most effective and reliable solution for CBPP surveillance. However, the final diagnosis of CBPP has to be confirmed by culture of the agent from lung tissue.

The pilot study concentrated on abattoirs with more than 300 cattle slaughtered per year, representing more than 87% of the whole slaughter cattle population. The response rate of meat inspectors invited to participate in the study was 82%. During the study period, the detection rate was approximately 1 case per 2'600 adult cattle inspected (<0.1%). The geographical distribution of the cases was correlated with the cattle population and slaughter house density in the country. Most of the lungs forwarded for bacteriological examination showed the typical lesions as they had been described to the meat inspectors. *M. mycoides subsp. mycoides* SC could not be cultured from any of these samples, and the histopathological picture did not reveal any suspicion of CBPP. On the other hand, other *Mycoplasma sp.*, principally *M. bovis*, could be isolated. This finding was surprising, because such isolations out of lung tissue have never been made in Switzerland.

Despite the lack of culture of the aetiological agent, some pathologically suspicious cases were traced back to their herds of origin, and blood samples taken from these animals. The sera were tested for anti-CBPP antibodies. 98.4% gave negative results, and 1.6% reacted positively, with titers no higher than 1/10+++. Such low titers have been observed in CBPP affected individuals, but Santini (personal communications, 1993) reported that in infected herds, titers higher than 1/160 are regularly observed. On the other hand, it is generally accepted that the CF-test used lacks good specificity, and commonly gives false positive reactions. These results showed that the characteristic pathological picture of CBPP can hardly be called pathognomic, and that other agents may provoke similar lesions, particularly the 'marble lung'. Nevertheless, the sensitivity of a surveillance system based on the examination of altered lungs can still be considered to be more sensitive than alternative methods, because these lungs are high-risk indicators. Furthermore, random sampling of inconspicuous lungs did not provide any additional information, and is besides much more complicated to integrate into the routine meat inspection procedure.

The organization and conduct of a CBPP surveillance system in slaughterhouses turned out to be not too difficult. The motivation of the meat inspectors was improved by personal contact, well designed information material and immediate feedback of results. To reduce extra work and cost for the abattoirs, they were provided with sampling material, and free mailing slips. The high quality samples turned in proved the good response of the people involved at the slaughter lines.

For the reasons stated above, the CBPP surveillance system based on slaughterhouse observations, as it has been designed in the pilot study, is considered to be the most practical and most reliable data source to document the absence of CBPP in Switzerland. Based on such data, there is no evidence of the occurrence of CBPP in this country. However, due to the short time period covered so far by the pilot study, a seasonal variation cannot be excluded.

This system will be recommended for continued routine CBPP surveillance in Switzerland as a supplement to the regular reporting system of clinical signs of the disease. It may also serve as a model for other countries.

REFERENCES

Etheridge, J.R., Cottew, S.D. and Lloyd, L.C. (1976): Studies on the origin of false positive reactions to the complement fixation test for contagious bovine pleuropneumonia. Austral. Vet. J. 52, 299-304.

ter Laak, E.A. (1992): Contagious bovine pleuropneumonia - A review. Vet. Quart. 15, 104-110.

O.I.E. (1989): Report of the Expert Consultation on Rinderpest Surveillance Systems. Office International des Epizooties, Paris.

O.I.E. (1992): Manual of standards for diagnostic tests and vaccines for List A and B diseases of mammals, birds and bees. Office International des Epizooties, Paris.

O.I.E. (1993): Report of the *Ad Hoc* Group on Contagious Bovine Pleuropneumonia (CBPP) Surveillance Systems. (unpublished).

Poumarat, F., Perrin, M., Belli, P., Longchamp, D., Le Goffe, C. and Martel, J.L. (1989): Recherche sur l'origine des fausses réactions positives dans le diagnostic sérologique de la péripneumonie contagieuse bovine. Revue Elev. Méd. vét. Pays trop. 42, 371-378.

Provost, A., Perreau, P., Bréard, A., Le Goff, C., Martel, J.L. and Cottew, G.S. (1987): Contagious bovine pleuropneumonia. Rev. sci. tech. Off. int. Epiz. 6, 625-679.

Regalla, J., Tavares, A,. Albuquerque, T., Cruz, E., Sereno, R. and Oliveira, J. (1990): Some epidemiological aspects of contagious bovine pleuropneumonia in Portugal (1983-1988) with reference to the incidence of cross-reations due to other Mycoplasma species isolated from bovines. In: Contagious bovine pleuropneumonia, J. Regalla (ed.), CEC publication EUR 12065 EN, Luxembourg, pp. 64-79.

PRELIMINARY FINDINGS FROM A BOVINE MORTALITY SURVEY

F.D. MENZIES*, T.D.G. BRYSON*, T. McCALLION** and D.I. MATTHEWS**

Measures for the prevention and control of disease are an important component of any profitable livestock production system Hence, accurate estimations of the number of bovine mortalities and assessment of the relative importance of various disease syndromes in such deaths are important in promoting cattle health within a country. When such information is available then the most appropriate advice on disease prevention and control can be provided to producers and areas requiring further research and development can be effectively targeted.

Cattle are very important to the Northern Ireland agri-food industry with over 1.5 million animals located on almost 90% of the 29,000 farms in the province. The average size of dairy cow and suckler cow herds in Northern Ireland are 41 and 15 cows respectively (Department of Agriculture for Northern Ireland, 1992).

The Veterinary Sciences Division (VSD) of the Department of Agriculture for Northern Ireland (DANI) operates a farm animal disease diagnostic service to the agricultural community through private veterinary practitioners. However, a relatively small proportion of total bovine mortalities are submitted to the VSD for post-mortem examination and there is a selection bias associated with these submissions.

A survey of bovine mortalities was carried out during 1992. The aims of this survey were to determine the number of mortalities occurring in various age groups and animal types and to determine the relative importance of various disease syndromes which contribute to bovine mortality during the year. The findings of the survey are described below.

METHODS

Producers to be included in the sample were drawn from the June 1991 Northern Ireland Agricultural Census. All farms which had more than 29 suckler cows or more than 69 dairy cows were included in the sample and the remainder of farms with cattle were sampled at a rate of 5%. The 4,395 farms in the sample contained 38% of total cattle in the province.

The questionnaire was pre-tested on a small number of producers. Four mailings were sent out to the producers over the duration of the survey. The final mailing in January 1993 included an additional form allowing farmers who had no deaths over 1992 to record this fact. Producers were also given the opportunity to withdraw from the survey at any stage by

*Veterinary Sciences Division, Stormont, Stoney Road, Belfast BT4 3SD
**Biometrics Division, Newforge Lane, Belfast BT9 5PX

returning the cover letter using the pre-paid envelopes provided.

The validity of the questionnaires was checked by visual assessment and by various computerised cross-checks which were performed while the data were being entered into a SPSS-X systems file. SPSS-X was the main software package used for statistical analysis of the data.

Notifiable diseases

Cattle sent for casualty slaughter were included as bovine mortalities but animals slaughtered as a result of notifiable diseases were excluded from the analysis. Numbers of cattle slaughtered through having a notifiable disease or being in-contacts are already known from data collected by DANI Veterinary Service.

RESULTS

The overall response rate from farmers was 29.7%, with response rates being very similar over the different categories of herd type and size. Information was provided by 1,306 producers reported over 3,500 bovine mortalities during 1992. Some reasons given for non-participation included retirement or death of the farmer or that the farmer felt that his herd was too small to be of any use to the survey. The majority of non-participants did not give a reason.

The estimated total number of cattle deaths in Northern Ireland during 1992 was 23,100 (this figure excludes 7,900 estimated stillbirths). This is comprised of 4,250 dairy cow deaths, 6,000 suckler cow deaths and 12,350 deaths in young stock. The overall annual mortality rate was estimated to be 2.0%. If stillbirths were excluded, the overall estimated mortality rate was 1.5%. Table 1 details the annual mortality rates for each animal type.

Smaller herds showed consistently higher mortality rates in all animal types. This difference was statistically significant for suckler cows and for 6-24 month old cattle.

Over 3,000 of the mortalities recorded were from farms with larger herds, that is, more than 69 dairy cows or more than 29 suckler cows. Only the data relating to the strata for these larger farms were used in the following analyses.

Table 2 illustrates the seasonal pattern of mortalities by each animal type. Overall, March-April were the months in which highest mortality rates were encountered. In suckler cows, March-May and September-October were the months of highest mortality while January-May was the period in which the majority (59%) of dairy cows died. In calves under one month old, one-third of mortalities occurred in March-April which was also the period in which the largest proportion of mortalities occurred in 6-24 month old cattle. The months of December and January accounted for 23% of 1-5 month old calf mortalities.

One-third of suckler cows were found dead without any previous signs of illness being noticed. Recumbency (18%), convulsions (11%) and ill-thrift (11%) were also common clinical signs preceding suckler cow deaths.

Table 1. Estimated annual mortality rates by animal type in Northern Ireland during 1992.

Animal Type	**Annual mortality rate (%)**
Suckler cows	2.36
Dairy cows	1.55
Stillbirths	1.86[a]
Under 1 month old	1.02[a]
1-5 months	0.82[a]
6 to 24 months old	0.79
Over 24 months (excluding cows)	0.29

[a]The annual mortality rate for calves under six months old was calculated using the estimated number of deaths as the numerator and the number of cattle under one year old as the denominator.

Table 2. Seasonal percentage mortality by animal type for bovine mortalities in Northern Ireland during 1992.

Season	**Suckler Cow**	**Dairy Cow**	**Under 1mth**	**1-5 mths**	**6-24mths**	**Overall**
Jan-Mar	23.9	37.4	35.1	24.4	26.1	31.2
Apr-Jun	32.6	28.3	28.1	30.5	27.1	29.0
Jul-Sep	21.5	10.9	11.3	21.9	22.6	15.5
Oct-Dec	22.0	23.4	25.5	23.2	24.2	24.3
% of deaths	19.3	14.4	45.6	11.2	8.8	99.3[a]

[a]0.7% of deaths were bulls and fatstock over two years old.

Recumbency (24%) was the main sign associated with dairy cow mortalities. Mastitis (18%) also accounted for a high proportion of dairy cow deaths and eleven per cent of recumbent dairy cows also had mastitis. Dairy cows which were found dead were also a common occurrence (19% of all dairy cow mortalities).

The majority of deaths in calves under one month old presented as stillbirths (62%). Diarrhoea (19%) was the main clinical sign in those born alive. When stillbirths were excluded, diarrhoea was associated with almost half (48%) of the mortalities in this young age group.

Pneumonia was the dominant clinical sign in mortalities amongst 1-5 month and 6-24 month age groups.

Approximately 75% of all cattle in which clinical signs were observed prior to death or which were sent for casualty slaughter, were examined by a veterinary surgeon. An exception was in neonatal calves where only 46% received veterinary attention (only 21% of stillbirths were attended by a veterinary surgeon).

Veterinary diagnoses were grouped for each animal type depending on the main system or syndrome involved (Table 3). Perinatal conditions (conditions associated with calving) were the main cause of mortality in both dairy and suckler cows. The main perinatal conditions relating to suckler cow deaths were metritis and downer cow syndrome which were also major causes of mortality in dairy cows together with nerve paralysis and post-partum haemorrhage. Diseases of the central nervous system (22%) were major causes of death in suckler cows while mastitis contributed to 17% of dairy cow deaths. Gastro-intestinal problems caused most mortalities in neonatal calves while respiratory diseases were the major cause of mortalities in older cattle.

Table 3. Combined veterinary diagnoses by system affected or syndrome for each animal type for bovine mortalities in Northern Ireland during 1992.

System/ Syndrome	Suckler Cow (%)	Dairy Cow (%)	Under 1 mth (%)	1-5 months (%)	6-24 months (%)	Total (%)
Perinatal/ Genital	29.1	30.8	n/a	n/a	2.5	13.3
GI Tract	9.5	13.0	26.1	32.6	21.7	19.9
Respiratory	2.0	2.9	10.6	37.4	36.9	14.0
Mastitis	10.8	17.0	n/a	n/a	0.0	6.0
Central nervous	22.0	4.3	5.2	3.7	3.8	8.3
Locomotor	7.4	11.6	3.4	8.4	19.1	8.9
Stillbirths	n/a	n/a	47.5	n/a	n/a	13.9
Miscellaneous	19.2	20.4	7.2	17.9	16.0	15.7
Number of deaths	296	276	387	190	157	1320[a]
% of deaths	22.4	20.9	29.3	14.4	11.9	98.9[a]

[a]14 deaths (1.1% of total mortalities) were bulls and fatstock over two years old.

No specific condition predominated among the perinatal deaths in dairy and suckler cows although 8% of suckler cows were diagnosed as dying from metritis. 20% of suckler cow mortalities which were examined ante-mortem by a veterinary surgeon died from hypomagnesaemia. Coliform mastitis (12%) was the main specific diagnosis associated with dairy cow mortalities and also accounted for 7% of suckler cow deaths. Thirty-four per cent of mortalities in calves under one month were associated with dystokia while undifferentiated scours (11%) and pneumonia of undefined aetiology (10%) were the main causes of mortality in neonatal calves. Pneumonia of undefined aetiology (31%) was the predominant cause of mortality in 1-5 month old calves and also in 6-24 month old cattle although the proportion fell to 26% of calf mortalities in the older age group. Bovine viral diarrhoea/mucosal disease (BVD/MD) and blackleg were also significant causes of mortality in young stock and were associated with between 5% and 10% of deaths in these age groups.

A concurrent survey of veterinary practices confirmed the above findings in relation to the major causes of mortality by each animal type.

DISCUSSION

The response rate of almost 30% was considered satisfactory for a postal survey. The number of returns has enabled estimations of the number of mortalities within the different animal types and has also allowed the identification of the most important disease syndromes within each group.

The mortality rates reported in the present study were lower than those recorded in other countries. For instance, the mortality rate in dairy cows in Denmark has varied between 3.5% and 4.2% over the last decade (Agger and Willeberg, 1991). In California, the estimated mortality rate was 2.0% in dairy cows, 1.2% in young stock and approximately 2.7% in unweaned dairy calves (Gardner et al., 1990). A study on Ontario dairy farms indicated mortality rates of between 3.9% and 6.7% in unweaned heifer calves (Waltner-Toews et al., 1986). Suckler calf mortality rates of between 3% and 6% have been recorded in Great Britain (Meat and Livestock Commission, 1987) and average mortality rates in range calves in the U.S.A. were 6.7% (Patterson et al., 1987). In a survey of livestock diseases carried out in Northern Ireland during 1954/55, mortality rates of 1.2% for cows, 1.7% for heifer and steers and 2.8% for calves under six months of age were found (Gracey, 1960).

The present survey consistently identified a higher mortality rate in smaller herds. One or more of the following hypotheses might be advanced to explain this:-

a) There are a higher proportion of smaller herds in the less favoured areas. Such herds are under increased nutritional and environmental stress.
b) Many owners of smaller cattle herds are part-time farmers and therefore spend less time observing and attending to their cattle.
c) Some owners of smaller herds may have only limited experience and training in animal health.

The seasonal pattern of cow mortalities tends to be mainly related to the months in which most calves are born (March-May). A second peak in suckler cow mortalities in September-October occurs during one of the known high risk periods for hypomagnesaemia (grass tetany). Obviously, stillbirths and neonatal calf mortalities are also closely related to the calving pattern. The majority of mortalities in older calves tended to occur throughout the period when young stock are normally housed.

A high proportion of suckler cows (33%) were found dead with a significant number of these deaths occurring during the autumn. The apparently short period of illness before death and the time of year at which most occurred would suggest that a significant number of these suckler cow mortalities could be due to hypomagnesaemia. This hypothesis is supported by the fact that over 20% of suckler cow deaths in which veterinary attention was received ante-mortem were diagnosed as having hypomagnesaemia and that convulsions was one of the main clinical signs reported by farmers. The majority of dairy cow deaths in which no clinical signs were observed ante-mortem also occurred during the recognised danger periods for hypomagnesaemia. Reduction in the number of mortalities from grass tetany could be achieved by ensuring that cows receive an adequate daily intake of magnesium (30g) particularly during the spring and autumn. Standard methods of supplementing dietary magnesium are well documented elsewhere (McCoy, 1993).

Recumbency was the main clinical sign recorded in suckler and dairy cows but little can be determined directly from this information as recumbency is a non-specific clinical sign. This is also the case with ill-thrift.

Mastitis was cited in 18% of all dairy cow deaths. Coliform mastitis caused 12% of all mortalities in dairy cows receiving veterinary attention as well as 7% of suckler cow deaths which received veterinary treatment. Coliform mastitis is an environmental mastitis which occurs shortly after calving. Measures to reduce the incidence of these infections would include improving hygiene around calving, ensuring clean, dry bedding and appropriate cubicle design.

Approximately 30% of all suckler and dairy cows die or are sent for casualty slaughter because of injuries or conditions related to calving. These losses could be reduced by ensuring the use of bulls known to produce progeny which are of moderate birth weight, ensuring that cows are at their recommended condition score at calving and by farmers receiving adequate training in basic obstetrics. The choice of appropriate bull is particularly important in relation to breeding heifers.

A significant proportion of mortalities were due to stillbirth (20% of the total bovine mortalities and 62% of mortalities in calves under one month old). Dystokia (difficulty in calving) was involved in the great majority (71%) of the stillbirths where a veterinary surgeon was in attendance although, veterinary assistance was only sought in 21% of all stillbirths. Increased supervision and proper management at calving and selection of sires which are known to have fewer calving problems are areas which should be considered if losses due to stillbirths are to be reduced.

Diarrhoea accounted for 48% of all neonatal mortalities. Overall, the "neonatal disease complex" was the cause of death in the majority of young calves reflecting similar findings in other studies (Meat and Livestock Commission, 1986; Bakheit and Green, 1981). Reduction in the number of mortalities from this disease complex could be achieved by ensuring that new-born calves receive adequate colostrum shortly after birth, strategic vaccination of the dam against Rotavirus/K99 *E. coli* and ensuring calving areas and calf rearing areas are clean, dry and warm. Young calves should also be kept separate from older calves. Only 46% of this group received any veterinary attention, therefore there is also scope for better therapy and nursing care which could be provided by a greater veterinary input. In suckler cows, management of the herd to allow a compact calving pattern could help reduce the number of calf mortalities as many calves born late in the calving season succumb to disease because of gradual build up of infectious agents in the environment over the calving season (Lowman, 1988).

Control of infectious pneumonias in young calves is greatly assisted by providing good housing, particularly adequate ventilation, a dry bed and avoidance of drafts at stock level. Whenever possible, calves of similar age should be reared in self-contained groups of 30 calves or less and an all-in, all-out system operated. Although vaccines currently available do not provide satisfactory control of pneumonia in all age groups, their use under veterinary direction may be beneficial in certain situations. Prompt veterinary treatment is essential in severe outbreaks of pneumonia.

BVD/MD was a relatively important cause of death in young stock. BVD/MD could also be responsible for a proportion of the stillbirths. Specific farms usually have an identified BVD problem. This disease can be eliminated by detection and elimination of animals persistently infected with BVD virus although this approach may cause severe problems if infection regained entry to a totally susceptible herd.

Although blackleg is a disease which is easily prevented by use of very effective and relatively cheap vaccines, approximately 5% of calf deaths are caused by this condition.

This survey has highlighted the major causes of bovine mortality in Northern Ireland and has identified important conditions for which the application of preventative measures, including attention to management, could significantly reduce the number of avoidable cattle deaths.

CONCLUSIONS

An estimated 23,100 cattle died on farms in Northern Ireland during 1992. These deaths included 4,250 dairy cows and 6,000 suckler cows. Almost one-third of cow mortalities were associated with perinatal conditions. The most commonly identified causes of mortalities within each bovine type were hypomagnesaemia in suckler cows, coliform mastitis in dairy cows and diarrhoea and pneumonia in younger stock. There were also 7,900 stillbirths reported. The overall annual cost to the cattle industry from these mortalities is estimated to be almost £11,000,000.

This survey permits quantification of the number of mortalities occurring in various groups and the relative importance of various disease syndromes associated with bovine mortalities during 1992. The information forms a useful base for advice on prevention of these important cattle diseases. It also highlights the need for continuing research work in such areas as stillbirths, perinatal conditions in cows, pneumonia, scours and coliform mastitis so that effective control strategies can be devised.

REFERENCES

Agger, J.F. and Willeberg, P. (1991) Production and mortality in dairy cows from 1960-1990: time series analysis of ecological data. Proceedings of the 6th ISVEE Symposium. Ottawa: International Symposium on Veterinary Epidemiology and Economics. 357-360 pp.

Bakheit, H.A. and Green, H.J. (1981) Control of bovine neonatal diarrhoea by management techniques. Vet. Rec. 108, 55-458.

Department of Agriculture for Northern Ireland (1992) Statistical review of Northern Ireland agriculture. D.A.N.I. publication. 45-46 pp.

Gardner, I.A., Hird, D.W., Utterback, W.W., Danaye-Elmi, C., Heron, B.R., Christiansen, K.H. and Sischo, W.H. (1990) Mortality, morbidity, case-fatality, and culling rates for Californian dairy cattle as evaluated by the National Animal Health Monitoring System, 1986-87. Prev. Vet. Med. 8, 157-170.

Gracey, J.F. (1960) Survey of livestock diseases in Northern Ireland. H.M.S.O., Belfast. 59 p.

Lowman, B.G. (1988) Suckler cow management. In Pract. 10, 91-100.

McCoy, M.A. (1993) Grass tetany in Northern Ireland. Agric. in N. Ireland. 7(3), 12-13.

Meat and Livestock Commission (1986) Veterinary aspects of beef production - calf disease and mortality. In: Beef Yearbook 1986. Bletchley, England: M.L.C.. 89-91 pp.

Meat and Livestock Commission (1987) Beefplan results - Suckler beef systems. In: Beef Yearbook 1987. Bletchley, England: M.L.C. 49-61 pp.

Patterson, D.J., Bellows, R.A., Burfening, P.J. and Carr, J.B. (1987) Occurrence of neonatal and post-natal mortality in range calves. Theriogen. 28, 557-571.

Waltner-Toews, D., Martin, S.W., Meek, A.H. and McMillan, I. (1986) Dairy calf management, morbidity and mortality in Ontario Holstein herds. The data. Prev. Vet. Med. 4, 103-124.

POULTRY EPIDEMIOLOGY

THE EPIDEMIOLOGY AND CONTROL OF ECONOMICALLY IMPORTANT DISEASES OF BROILER AND BROILER BREEDER PRODUCTION

S G McILROY*

World production of poultry meat represents approximately 23% of all meat production and is increasing annually. During the past 25 years world poultry meat production and consumption has trebled with higher production (20.6 kilograms per head) in countries with a developed market economy than production (3.6 kilogram per head) in those countries with a developing market economy. The United Kingdom (UK) is currently the seventh major producer of poultry meat and the annual gross output from poultry meat production in the UK is valued at approximately £900 million (FAO, 1992).

Important factors in the growth of the poultry industry in developed countries are the efficiency of poultry in converting vegetable protein into animal protein, the attractiveness and aesthetic acceptability of poultry meat to consumers and the highly competitive costs of production. The increased size of the poultry meat industry, to satisfy increased consumer demand, has been made possible by the introduction of intensive production systems utilising new technologies. The UK poultry meat industry is concentrated in less than twenty large integrated organisations most of which have control of broiler parent flocks, hatcheries, as well as the broiler generation production. Most integrations also control the processing of the final broiler product. Effective disease control at all levels in such intricate, integrated organisations has been an essential component of the growth and economic success of the industry (Law & Payne, 1990).

Numerous attempts have been made to estimate the economic losses caused by disease in poultry meat production. In general, the prevalence and severity of disease, both viral and bacterial, is greater in developing countries where management systems are often less intensive and less well controlled. In the UK mortality has been estimated to cause a minimum loss of 7% of the value of the industry, while the inclusion of losses due to reduced productivity, condemnations and the cost of prophylaxis and treatment has been estimated to increase the overall losses to approximately 20% (Biggs, 1982). However, a wide range in the prevalence and severity of disease between individual flocks and between poultry organisations is common and therefore the opportunity for effective disease control to substantially reduce the overall cost of poultry meat production is always present (Jones et al.,1978).

*Ross Breeders Ltd, Newbridge, Midlothian EH28 8SZ, Scotland

Furthermore, new diseases such as Egg Drop Syndrome, Chicken Anaemia Agent, Turkey Rhinotracheitis and Big Liver and Spleen Disease, or more virulent strains of endemic diseases such as very virulent Marek's disease, virulent Infectious Bursal disease and variant pathogenic Infectious Bronchitis viruses, may not be controlled by existing procedures such as currently available vaccines. (McNulty, 1993). Under these circumstances disease can cause catastrophic losses to the industry.

INFECTIOUS BRONCHITIS

Epidemiology

Cause: Infectious bronchitis (IB) was first described in the USA in 1931 as a highly contagious respiratory disease of chickens. It now has a world-wide distribution. The causal organism is a single stranded RNA virus of the family Coronoviridae. A number of antigenically different serotypes are recognised by virus neutralisation tests but all possess a common group antigen demonstrable by agar gel precipitation, immuno-fluorescence tests or ELISA. Common serotypes such as Massachusetts and Connecticut show a proclivity for the respiratory tract while some serotypes such as Gray and Holte are nephrotrophic. Variation in virulence occurs among isolates of the infectious bronchitis virus and new variant serotypes of variable pathogenicity can occur sporadically and may cause disease problems in areas where IB was previously effectively controlled by vaccination.

Spread of Infection: Direct airborne transmission of the virus from the respiratory tract between individual birds within a flock and between flocks is the commonest method of spread and can occur over large distances. Transmission through infected faeces can also occur. Vertical transmission has not been demonstrated under both experimental or field conditions (King & Cavanagh, 1991)

Economic Effects on Production

Infection may be asymptomatic or may result in clinical signs which reflect disease of the respiratory, renal or reproductive systems. The respiratory syndrome is the most common clinical manifestation in birds of all ages. Mortality in broilers or young breeders can be up to 25% if secondary bacterial or viral infections such as Escherichiae coli, Newcastle Disease or Turkey Rhinotracheitis Virus (TRT) are present. Poor growth and loss of uniformity can also occur. Similar levels of mortaltiy can be seen in young birds with the renal form of the disease. Mortality does not normally occur in adult birds. However, a recent variant serotype in the UK (Variant 793B) has been associated with myopathy, especially of the deep pectoral muscle and a variable mortality in breeders (Parsons et al., 1992). This variant has also been associated with a severe respiratory syndrome in broilers in the UK often with concurrent TRT and/or Escherichiae coli infections.

The reproductive syndrome is manifested by reduced egg production and poor quality of eggs. Egg production is usually reduced by between 5-10% but can be up to 50% if flocks are affected at peak production and thus within the period of maximum stress. Concurrent infection with TRT in breeders will increase the severity of the drop in egg production. Production may not return to normal levels for 4-6 weeks and the internal and external quality of the eggs produced can be severely affected. Poor quality eggs from affected flocks have a reduced hatchability and can also result in a reduced chick viability due to bacterial contamination through the thin and less effective shell defence structure.

Control and Prevention

Infectious bronchitis virus is ubiquitous in many regions and airborne transmission can occur over considerable distances. Thus, maintaining flocks free from infection may not be possible and control is normally based on increasing the resistance of the bird by vaccination, using attenuated strains. Control in breeders is normally affected by the routine use of both live and killed vaccines. Live vaccines are administered via the drinking water frequently at 3 and 8 weeks of age and a killed vaccine administered at between 16 and 18 weeks of age. In areas with an anticipated field challenge at an early age live vaccination at day old is common. This vaccination strategy has two objectives. The primary objective of the vaccination is to provide protection from an appropriate age to the young broiler breeder and thus reduce the adverse affects of field infection on subsequent breeder performance. The second objective is to produce high and uniform levels of maternal antibody to passively protect the progeny. In broilers, a live highly attenuated IB vaccine is usually administered via a coarse spray at day old to stimulate local immunity. In areas of high field challenge, IB vaccination is repeated at 18-21 days (Pattison, 1990). Most vaccinations are based on the Massachusetts serotype and give protection to a range of field isolates of different serotypes. However, Massachusetts vaccinated flocks may not be adequately protected against all serotypes and in many countries live and inactivated vaccines containing multiple serotypes are used. If available vaccines do not contain serotypes which are protective against a pathogenic variant, revaccination in breeders every 6-8 weeks with a Massachusetts based live vaccine throughout the production period has been used to stimulate local immunity. Local immunity is less specific than humoral antibody response and will provide protection against a wider range of antigens. This strategy is currently in operation in several European countries in an attempt to protect flock performance against the new variant serotype (793B) which at present is not included in any commercial live or killed vaccines.

NEWCASTLE DISEASE

Epidemiology

Cause: Newcastle Disease (ND) is caused by a group of closely related viruses which form the avian paramyxovirus type 1 serotype. Since the first recognition of Newcastle Disease in 1926, it has been reported from virtually every country and is regarded as being endemic in many countries. Vaccination against Newcastle

Disease is practised in all but a few of the countries producing poultry meat on a commercial scale, Northern Ireland, Republic of Ireland and Denmark being notable exceptions within the European Community. There are many different strains and serotypes of Newcastle Disease virus and categorisation of isolates has been used epidemiologically to monitor epizootics such as the pigeon associated Newcastle Disease outbreaks which appeared throughout the world during the 1980s. Many Newcastle Disease isolates cause distinctive clinical signs and severity of disease, including mortality, and have been categorised into five pathotypes. These categories are viscerotropic velogenic, neurotropic velogenic, mesogenic, lentogenic respiratory and asymptomatic enteric Newcastle Disease viruses.

Newcastle Disease is a notifiable disease in most countries of the world. It is now accepted for international control and trade certification that a Newcastle Disease outbreak is any infection by an avian PMV1 with an intracerebral pathogenicity index (ICPI) of over 0.7 (McCracken et al., 1992).

Spread of infection: The spread of ND virus is highly dependent on the organ in which the particular virus multiplies. Thus, ND virus isolates which multiple in the respiratory tract spread rapidly between individuals in a flock and usually between flocks in an area. Isolates that are mainly restricted to intestinal replication may spread slowly between individual birds and less predictably between flocks in an area. Racing pigeons and trade in exotic birds have been responsible for panzootic spread of ND virus, while the contamination of poultry feed has been implicated in epidemics in several EC countries (McCracken et al., 1992).

Economic Effects on Production

The severity of the disease produced following infection with ND virus will vary depending on the virulence of the infecting virus and the age, health status and immune competence of the bird. The economic effects on breeder production will therefore vary from high mortality (up to 100%), high morbidity, exhibited by respiratory and nervous symptoms, and a severe drop in egg production (production can stop completely); to a mild and transient respiratory distress with slight (1-2%) drop in egg production. Broilers show a similar variability in the severity of clinical signs with mortality and respiratory symptoms predominating. Food conversion, weight and uniformity can be substantially affected.

However, the economic significance of ND to the poultry industry is not restricted to reduce performance in individual flocks but related to international control procedures which govern the definition of a disease outbreak (ICPI over 0.7) and the subsequent designation of a region's health status with regard to international trade in poultry and poultry products. Furthermore, many countries, such as the United Kingdom, have a compulsory slaughter policy for Newcastle Disease affected flocks. Newcastle Disease outbreaks can therefore cause very substantial economic losses to the poultry meat industry, independent of the effect on efficiency of production in individual broiler or breeder flocks.

Control and Prevention

Most countries have legislation to prevent the introduction of disease by infected birds or contaminated produce. Control procedures have evolved from epidemiological observations of the spread of the disease throughout the world and many countries have quarantine requirements for exotic birds and restrictions on the movement of racing pigeons, and compulsory vaccination of such birds. Most countries also have legislation to control ND outbreaks such as compulsory slaughter and obligatory ring vaccination following an outbreak. Some countries also have a compulsory routine vaccination programme for all flocks.

Vaccination of broiler breeders against ND is practised in most countries of the world even when no outbreaks with an ICPI greater than 0.7 have been identified. Three basic categories of ND vaccines are available. Live lentogenic vaccines are derived from field isolates with low pathogenicity. Examples are Hitchner B1 and La Sota. They are the least attenuated of the ND vaccines but have been selected to improve their immunogenicity. Cloning of the original isolates has also been used to decrease pathogenicity and enhance the immunogenicity of lentogenic vaccines. Other ND live vaccines are derived in the laboratory from fully virulent field isolates and are defined as Mesongenic vaccines. Mesogenic vaccines can produce a very high immune response but can cause severe disease and must only be administered after priming with live lentogenic vaccine. Mesogenic vaccines are prohibited in many countries and their use is restricted to regions with endemic velogenic field strains, such as the Middle East.

Inactivated ND vaccines are also used to control ND. Both virulent and avirulent isolates have been used to produce the killed antigen and oil or aqueous based injections are administered intramuscularly. Inactivated vaccines are commonly used at 16-18 weeks in breeders following initial priming with live vaccines to produce high and uniform humoral antibody levels in a similar manner to IB vaccination programmes. Such antibody titres are considered protective during the production period. Furthermore, high and uniform levels of maternal antibody are considered desirable to protect the broiler progeny from ND virus. In regions with ND outbreaks, revaccination during the production period with live lentogenic vaccines may be carried out to stimulate local immunity and enhance the immuno-competence of the bird to anticipated virulent field infections.

AVIAN INFLUENZA

Epidemiology

Cause: Avian influenza (AI) is a disease syndrome caused by any type A influenza virus, a member of Orthomyxoviridae family. The disease was first described in Italy in 1878 with very high mortality in chickens and became known as Fowl Plague. There are a very large number of subtypes within the influenza type A viruses and these are determined by the expression of two major surface protein antigens, haemagglutinin (H) and neuraminidase (N). There are currently 13 recognised H subtypes and 9 N subtypes. Each virus expresses one H and one N subtype and most of the 117 possible combinations have been identified. Certain H subtypes have been associated with high pathogenicity and to date all highly pathogenic H subtypes have been either 7 or 5. The major epidemiological features of influenza viruses are their large natural reservoir in wild birds, their ability to cross between different host species, the potential variable expression of pathogenicity of the same subtype and the ability for recombination with other influenza viruses to produce new virus of different antigenic expression and pathogenicity. An example of the latter was seen in China when virus spread from wild fowl to domestic ducks, then to pigs and eventually to man causing the "Hong Kong" influenza panzootic of 1969 (Yasuda et al, 1991).

Spread of Infection: Influenza viruses replicate in the respiratory and intestinal tracts of infected birds and transmission is via direct contact with infected droplets or in faecal material. Spread within a population of birds is often relatively slow in both natural and experimental infections and it is estimated that the faecal oral route may be the normal mechanism of spread. Airborne transmission over large distances has not been observed and movement of personnel and fomites has been associated with the dessemination of the disease in most recorded outbreaks.

Economic Effects on Production

The economic effects of AI on production is highly variable and dependent on the pathogenicity of the virus and the age, health status and immunocompetence of the host. Highly pathogenic avian influenza (HPAI) viruses causing classical Fowl Plague result in very high mortality of over 50% and a severe drop in egg production in breeders. Clinical signs frequently reflect the target organ affected with acute enteric signs and respiratory involvement predominating. In broilers, mortality and reduced performance (food conversion and average weight) are the principle observed effects on production.

As with Newcastle Disease, the major impact of Avian Influenza on the modern broiler industry is not restricted to the reduced performance of individual broiler or breeder flocks but related to international control programmes which govern the definition of a disease outbreak and the designation of a regions health status with regard to international veterinary trade certification. Field isolates with an intravenous pathogenicity index (IVPI) of more than 1.2 are considered to be highly pathogenic avian influenza viruses. However, this criteria will not identify isolates that are ostensibly of low virulence but have the potential to mutate to an HPAI virus. Thus, amino acid sequencing of the haemagglutinin molecule in H5 and H7 serotypes is now carried out within the EC on influenza isolates to identify those with the potential for pathogenicity. The cost of the eradication of outbreaks of HPAI virus infections can be enormous to both government and the poultry meat industry. For example, the outbreaks in 1983 to 1984 in the USA cost the government over 60 million dollars while additional industry costs were estimated at 349 million dollars, most of which was passed on to the consumer. (Lasley, 1987)

Control and Prevention

Most countries have legislative control procedures that must be implemented following an outbreak of HPAI virus. Furthermore, all countries with developed poultry industries have policies aimed at preventing the introduction of HPAI viruses through trade with other countries and regions. In addition, eradication policies are normally applied if an outbreak occurs within a country. However, few countries have eradication schemes for influenza viruses of low virulence, but pathogenic potential, the EC member states being recent exceptions. Inactivated vaccines based on the H antigen have been used in some countries, such as the USA, to control the spread of influenza virus infections of lower pathogenicity than HPAI isolates. Live vaccines are not permitted because pathogenic strains may arise and there could be a risk of public health.

MAREK'S DISEASE

Epidemiology

Cause: Marek's disease (MD) is a lymphoproliferative disease of chickens caused by a herpesvirus. The disease is named after the Hungarian veterinarian who first described the condition in 1907. The disease has a worldwide distribution and was the most significant economic loss to the developing poultry industry prior to vaccines being available in the early 1970s. Three serotypes of MD virus and related herpesviruses have been defined. Serotype 1 comprises all oncogenic strains of MD virus and their derivatives. Serotype 1 field isolates have a range of virulence with some highly pathogenic isolates being termed very virulent Marek's disease viruses (VVMDV). Serotype 2 is a group of naturally apathogenic and non-oncogenic strains of MD virus and serotype 3 is an apathogenic and antigenically related herpesvirus of turkeys (HVT).

Spread of Infection: Marek's disease virus cannot be transmitted through the egg and therefore day old chicks are free of infection. Young chicks usually encounter the virus in their environment within the first few weeks of life. The virus is commonly present in poultry house dust and litter as a result of shedding of the virus from previous flocks. Infection is commonly airborne via the respiratory system. Within a few days the virus spreads, especially to lymphoid tissue where the characteristic lymphomatous changes occur. Within two weeks the virus spreads to the feather follicles where new infectious virus particles are formed and shed in large numbers in feather and skin debris into the environment throughout the life of the bird. Vaccinated birds will still become infected and shed the virus. The virus can survive in the poultry house environment for up to one year.

Economic Effects on Production

Marek's disease occurs in chickens from 6 weeks of age onwards, is most common between 12 and 24 weeks, but sometimes predominantly affects adult birds. Several forms of the disease occur. In affected breeder flocks, mortality is highly variable depending on the virulence of the strain but levels of between 10 - 30% are not uncommon. Egg production, hatchability and chick viability are usually not affected but poor chick quality from affected flocks has been reported in the UK and may be due to secondary infections. MD in broilers can affect mortality, food conversion, weight, yield and result in substantial levels of condemnations. In Europe, the disease is usually only apparent in broilers grown to heavier weights and over 60 days of age. However, the disease is common in the USA where broiler houses are not routinely cleaned out after each crop of birds. Recently, a new expression of the MD virus in broilers has been described in the UK as 'Floppy Broiler Syndrome' (Randall, Pers. Comm.). This condition is caused by MD virus infection of the brain and can occur in young broilers between 21 and 40 days of age. Gross pathological tumour lesions are not apparent and diagnosis is by histopathological examination only.

Prior to the availability of vaccines, condemnation rates due to MD lesions in broilers in the USA were on average 1.57% in 1970 and estimated to cost the industry over 200 million dollars at this time. Following the introduction of the HVT vaccines this condemnation rate reduced to 0.08% in 1982, a 95% reduction. (Payne, 1990).

Control and Prevention

There are no methods of treatment of Marek's disease and control is based on management methods which isolate young chicks from sources of infection, the use of genetically resistant stock and vaccination procedures. Some broiler breeds have been selected to increase genetic resistance to Marek's disease. For example, in the early 1980s Ross Breeders identified a genetic locus at the major histocompatability complex which was associated with a significantly increased susceptibility to mortality due to Marek's disease tumours. It was possible to demonstrate, using monoclonal antibodies, that the genetic locus was linked to the expression of a B blood group allele, the subtype 9. The B9 blood group subtype was present at frequencies of up to 20% in some genetic lines and this susceptible population of birds was removed from the breeding programme using a specific monoclonal antibody test. This strategy significantly increased the overall resistance of the Ross genotype to Marek's disease whilst ensuring that day old chicks can still adequately respond to appropriate vaccination strategies.

Commercially available vaccines have been derived from all three Marek's disease virus serotypes for use either alone or in combination. Serotype 1 vaccines are attenuated virulent or mildly virulent strains of MD virus. Examples are the UK derived HPRS 16 attenuated strain and the widely used CVI 988 (Rispens) strain from the Netherlands. Serotype 2 vaccines are derived from the apathogenic, non-oncogenic isolates and an example is the SB1 vaccine used in the USA. Serotype 3 vaccines are derived from the herpesvirus of turkeys (HVT). All three serotype vaccines are used in a cell associated form except HVT which can also be used as a cell free virus in a freeze dried form. Vaccine strategies for breeders include bivalent combinations at day old of HVT (serotype 3) and either SB1 (serotype 2) or Rispens/HPRS 16 (serotype 1) vaccines. Revaccination with freeze dried HVT at between 2 and 3 weeks of age is common in areas where very virulent Marek's disease virus is present. Day old vaccination in broilers, usually with HVT only, depends on the anticipated level and duration of environmental challenge. Thus, all broilers are routinely vaccinated in the USA, while broilers grown to heavy weights (greater than 2.5Kg) are routinely vaccinated in the UK and Italy.

SALMONELLOSIS

Epidemiology

Cause: Salmonella is a well defined genus in the family Enterobacteriaceae consisting of over 2,000 antigenically defined serotypes which are currently regarded as species. From the point of view of disease, the Salmonella serotypes can be divided into three major groups. The first group contains serotypes which characteristically produced systemic disease. The disease is frequently limited to the host species affected. Such serotypes include S. pullorum and S. gallinarum in chickens. These serotypes rarely produce human food poisoning. S. pullorum causes bacillary white diarrhoea or "pullorum" disease in young chicks. S. gallinarum is a highly pathogenic variant producing Fowl Typhoid in poultry of all ages.

The second group contains the vast majority of Salmonella serotypes many of which are frequently isolated from animal feeds and poultry. Most or all of these are able to produce human food poisoning but do not generally produce disease in poultry. The importance for poultry is thus related to their public health significance.

The third group comprises two serotypes, S. typhimurium and S. enteritidis which possess characteristics of both of the above groups. They are capable of producing systemic disease in young chickens, often with considerable mortality, but also produce the most severe form of food poisoning in man. (McIlroy et al., 1990).

Spread of Infection: All Salmonella colonise the intestinal tract and spread between birds is via the faecal oral route. Salmonella serotypes such as S. gallinarum, S. pullorum, S. enteritidis and S. typhimurium exhibit an affinity for poultry and are invasive. These serotypes can infect the reproductive tract and are vertically transmitted in the egg. The ability of a Salmonella serotype to exhibit true transovarian infection and thus invariable vertical transmission is the most important method of spread in the modern integrated poultry meat industry. Other serotypes can also spread vertically by faecal contamination of eggs but at a much reduced level and result in contamination of hatcheries and broiler progeny.

Feed stuffs can frequently become contaminated with Salmonella serotypes. The presence of animal proteins especially of poultry origin such as poultry offal meal and poultry feather meal in feed mills has been associated with the contamination of feed and resulted in the effective dissemination of Salmonella serotypes such as S. typhimurium, S. enteritidis, S. infantis, S. virchow and S. berta throughout and between integrated poultry organisations. Rodents, wild birds, contaminated water supply, humans, fomites etc can all be possible sources of Salmonella contamination for poultry flocks.

Economic Effects on Production

Broiler breeders are not normally affected clinically by the introduction of a Salmonella infection, although S. pullorum can cause substantial drops in egg production and morbidity. The major adverse economic effect of infection with other Salmonella serotypes in breeders is the possible dissemination to the hatchery and the day old broiler progeny. Both S. pullorum and S. gallinarum can cause high mortality, poor food conversion, decreased growth and yield, and substantial carcase condemnations due to septicaemic lesions. These substantial adverse effects on broiler performance are not normally observed with other Salmonella serotypes except S. enteritidis and occasionally some S. typhimurium phage types. Vertically transmitted S. enteritidis infection in broilers can cause mortality, morbidity and important economic losses from condemnations due to pericarditis and perihepatitis. (McIlroy et al., 1989)

The avian specific S. pullorum and S. gallinarum serotypes have been eradicated, using an agglutinating antibody test, from the intensive poultry industry in most of the countries with a developed market economy. They do not now constitute a significant economic loss. However, the economic loss to the industry from the other Salmonella serotypes is not restricted to reduced performance in broiler flocks. The economic loss to the industry from the presence of Salmonella serotypes is dictated by the possible occurrence of cases of human food poisoning due to the ingestion of contaminated poultry meat. Recent outbreaks in UK, Europe and USA due to S. enteritidis are causing concern to the industry. The extent of the present level of infection in poultry cannot be accurately assessed as it is constantly changing but poultry products are considered to be responsible for a significant number of human outbreaks of Salmonellosis in many countries. Although consumption of meat from diseased animals can give rise to food poisoning, the majority of cases of infected food are derived from healthy animals which are excreting small numbers of Salmonella in their faeces which cause cross infection and carcase contamination. Cross infection can result from stress factors, such as transport of chickens prior to slaughter, which increases the amount of Salmonella excreted. Carcase contamination can also follow slaughter. Use of scold tanks, de-feathering machines and chillers also increase carcase contamination levels resulting in up to 70% of poultry carcasses and up to 100% of giblet samples being contaminated.

Control and Prevention

Following the dramatic rise in the incidence of human food poisoning due to S. enteritidis and the increased isolation of the same phage type from poultry, a comprehensive national programme to control Salmonella infection in poultry was implemented in 1989 and a Codes of Practice for Poultry Flocks were issued jointly by MAFF and the British Poultry Federation. This has been superseded by an EC Zoonosis Directive from 1st January 1994 which harmonises the legislation and monitoring systems applied in all EC countries. Similar schemes are in operation in some states in the USA. Control is best achieved by preventing the introduction of Salmonella into flocks, especially breeder flocks, by using a series of biosecurity procedures such as decontaminated feed, rodent and wild bird control, isolation of sites and thorough cleansing and disinfection between flocks. A Government policy of compulsory slaughter with compensation for S. enteritidis infections in broiler breeder flocks was operated by several EC countries such as the UK and Holland. Antibiotic treatment, followed by the use of competitive exclusion products, has been advocated for the control of S. enteritidis infected broiler breeder flocks under the new EC Zoonosis Directive. Vaccines, both live and killed, are also under investigation for control of S. enteritidis infection in breeders. The ultimate assessment of the efficacy of any control procedure in S. enteritidis infected breeder flocks must be the blocking of vertical transmission via infected eggs and therefore the prevention of dissemination of the S. enteritidis serotype to hatcheries, broiler progeny, processing plants and ultimately the final consumer. This may require control strategies, in addition to procedures in the breeder flock, at multiple key locations in the process where the risk of contamination is high.

CHICKEN ANAEMIA AGENT

Epidemiology

Cause: Chicken Anaemia Agent (CAA) is an unclassified DNA virus with a single stranded, circular genome. CAA was first isolated in Japan in 1979. Experimentally, one day old chicks inoculated intramuscularly with the CAA agent developed severe anaemia, haemorrhages throughout the body, atrophy of the thymus and bursa of a Fabricius, yellowish bone marrow and liver changes (Yuasa, 1979). A similar disease known as Blue Wing or Anaemia Dermatitis Syndrome has been described under natural conditions both in layer and broiler chicks in many countries including Japan, Sweden, West Germany, USA, Great Britain and Northern Ireland (McIlroy et al., 1992).

Spread of Infection: The disease occurs in broiler flocks when in-lay broiler breeders with no previous exposure to the virus become infected. Under these conditions CAA is transmitted vertically in the egg to the broiler progeny which develop the disease from around 10-14 days of age. Serological studies have demonstrated that antibody to CAA is wide spread in commercial and SPF chickens world wide. It appears that in the United Kingdom most breeder flocks become infected before the laying period, presumably by ingestion of infected faeces from a small number of vertically infected birds, contamination of the flock by movement of personnel, fomites etc or from carry over of infection from previous breeder flocks. (McNulty et al., 1988). Thus outbreaks of clinical disease caused by CAA are relatively uncommon in the broiler progeny of breeder flocks (McIlroy et al., 1992). However, the broiler progeny of serologically positive breeders frequently develop antibodies to CAA in the absence of any clinical disease. This antibody presumably arises predominantly from horizontally acquired infection, either by ingestion of infected faeces from a small number of vertically infected broilers, contamination of the flock by personnel, fomites etc or from carry over of infection from previous broiler flocks (McNulty et al., 1991).

Economic Effects on Production

Clinical disease has only been observed in the progeny of breeder flocks which are sero-converting to CAA. Vertical transmission of CAA via the egg produces the characteristic Anaemia Dermatitis Syndrome between 10 and 28 days of age in the progeny. Vertical transmission to progeny occurs over a period of between 3-6 weeks and performance in the sero-converting breeder flocks is not affected. A variable mortality occurs in broilers which can reach 60% but usually averages 10%. The immuno-suppressive effects of CAA infection have been suggested to cause broilers to be highly susceptible to secondary bacterial infections. Average weight, uniformity and the overall economic performance are significantly reduced in affected broiler flocks (McIlroy et al., 1992) and this has been demonstrated using a computerised data retrieval system for broiler production data (McIlroy et al., 1988). This computer system has also qualified and quantified the significant adverse economic effects on production in commercial broiler flocks of subclinical CAA acquired by horizontal infection. Such horizontally acquired infections occur in over 50% of clinically normal broiler flocks in GB, Northern Ireland, Canada and probably many other countries (McNulty et al., 1991). The adverse economic effects of horizontally acquired subclinical infectious bursal disease have also been quantified in commercial broiler flocks using the computerised data retrieval system (McIlroy et al., 1989a).

Control and Prevention

Clinical disease due to CAA infection in broilers can be prevented by ensuring that breeder flocks have sero-converted before coming into lay. As reported, this normally occurs under field conditions in the UK. However, improved hygiene procedures in the UK and many other countries designed to maintain flocks free from Salmonella infections may increase the proportion of breeder flocks coming into lay without pervious exposure and thus increase the risk of clinical disease in the broiler progeny if exposure and sero-conversion occurs at a later stage. Live vaccines have been developed, some selected directly from field isolates and others attenuated through laboratory systems. CAA live vaccines for use in breeders are licensed in some countries and are currently being evaluated in the UK and therefore clinical CAA in broilers may be controlled relatively easily. However, the adverse economic effects of horizontally acquired, subclinical disease in broilers may be more important to the overall profitability of the broiler industry. Controlling such subclinical losses may be more difficult and require increasing the levels and uniformity of maternal antibody by the use of inactivated adjuvanted vaccines as have been developed for other avian diseases.

CONCLUSION

This paper has described the epidemiology and the economic effect of important diseases on both broiler and broiler breeder flock performace. The strategies utilised to prevent economic losses to the national and international poultry meat industry have been developed from those aspects of the epidemiology of each disease which facilitate effective control procedures. The extent and cost of control procedures must reflect the degree of economic loss from the disease.

The economic losses from a disease may not be limited to clinical signs. Substantial reductions in performance due to subclinical disease can occur and may only be quantified using data retrieval systems. Furthermore, the economical losses from reduced performance either clinical or subclinical in individual broiler or broiler breeder flocks may be inconsequential compared to those incurred from loss of trade and marketing when notifiable disease outbreaks are identified.

REFERENCES

Biggs, P.M. (1982). The world of poultry disease. Avian Pathol. II, 281-300.

F.A.O. (1992). 1991 FAO Production Year Book. Vol 45. Food and Agriculture Organisation of the United Nations, Rome.

Jones, H.G.R., Randall, C.R. and Hills, C.P.J. (1978). A survey of mortality in three adult broiler breeder flocks. Avian Pathol. 7, 619-628.

King, D.J. and Cavanagh, D (1991). Infectious Bronchitis. In; 'Diseases of Poultry'. Ed B.W. Calnek, Iowa State University press, Iowa, pp 471-484.

Lasley, F.A. (1987). Economics of avian influenza. Control vs noncontrol. Proc. 2nd Int. Symp. Avian Influenza. US Animal Health Assoc., Athens, pp 390-399.

Law, W.A. and Payne, L.N. (1990). The Poultry Industry. In; 'Poultry Diseases'. Ed. F.T.W. Jordan, Bailliere Tindall, London, pp 1-10.

McCracken, R.M., Denny, G.O. and MacDonald, S.C. (1992). Newcastle Disease - recent experiences during an outbreak in Northern Ireland. Proceedings of the Society of Veterinary Epidemiology and Preventive Medicine. 10, 40-46.

McIlroy, S.G., Goodall, E.A., Rainey, J. and McMurray, C.H. (1988). A computerised management and disease information retrieval system for profitable broiler production. Agric. Systems. 27, 11-22.

McIlroy, S.G., Goodall, E.A., and McCracken, R.M. (1989a). Economic effects of subclinical infectious bursal disease on broiler production. Avian Pathol. 18, 465-480.

McIlroy, S.G., McCracken, R.M., Neill, S.D. and O'Brien, J.J.(1989b). The control, prevention and eradication of Salmonella enteritidis infection in broiler and broiler breeder flocks. Vet. Rec. 125, 545-548.

McIlroy, S.G., Neill, S.D., Goodall, E.A., McLoughlin, E.M. and McCracken, R.M. (1990). Salmonella Isolates from Humans and Production Animal Species in Northern Ireland from 1979-1988. Society for Veterinary Epidemiology and Preventive Medicine. 8, 24-48.

McIlroy, S.G., McNulty, M.S., Bruce, D.W., Smyth, J.A., Goodall, E.A. and Alcorn, M.J. (1992). Economic effects of clinical chicken anaemia agent infection on profitable broiler production. Avian Dis. 36, 566-574.

McNulty, M.S., Connor, T.J., McNeilly, F., Kirkpatrick, M.S. and McFerran, J.B. (1988). A serological survey of domestic poultry in the United Kingdom for antibody to chicken anaemia agent. Avian Pathol. 17, 315-324.

McNulty, M.S., McIlroy, S.G., Bruce, D.W. and Todd, D. (1991). Economic effects of subclinical chicken anaemia agent infection in broiler chickens. Avian Dis. 35, 263-268.

McNulty, M.S. (1993). Recurrent and emerging diseases. Proc. Xth. International Congress of the World Vet. Poult. Assoc., pp 3-17.

Parsons, D., Ellis, M.M., Cavanagh, D. and Cook, J.K.A (1992). Characterisation of an infectious bronchitis virus isolated from vaccinated broiler breeder flocks. Vet. Rec. 131, pp 408-411.

Pattison, M (1990). Vaccines and Vaccination. In; 'Poultry Diseases'. Ed. F.T.W. Jordan, Balliere Tindall, London, pp 418-429.

Payne, L.N. (1990). Marek's Disease. In; 'Poultry Diseases' Ed. F.T.W. Jordan, Bailliere Tindall, London, pp 96-105.

Yasuda, J., Shortridge, K.F., Shimizu, Y. and Kida, F. (1991). Molecular evidence for a role of domestic ducks in the introduction of avian H3 influenza viruses to pigs in Southern China, where A/Hong Kong/68 (H3N2) strain emerged. Journ. of Gen. Virol. 72, 75-81.

Yuasa, N., Taniguchi, T. and Yoshida, I. (1979). Isolation and some characteristics of an agent inducing anaemia in chicks. Avian Dis. 23, 366-385.

A STRATEGY FOR DEALING WITH NEW VIRUS DISEASES OF POULTRY

M S McNULTY*

This paper outlines a strategy for dealing with new virus diseases of domestic poultry. The need for such a strategy becomes obvious when one considers the number of virus diseases that have been described in poultry over the last 15 years or so. These include egg drop syndrome, runting stunting syndrome, turkey rhinotracheitis/swollen head syndrome, hydropericardium syndrome, Newcastle disease caused by the pigeon variant of avian paramyxovirus type 1, big liver and spleen disease (reviewed by McNulty, 1993) and Muscovy duck parvovirosis (Fournier and Gaudry, 1994). Furthermore, changes in endemic virus diseases continue to pose problems. For example, antigenic and pathotypic variants of infectious bursal disease (IBD) virus have arisen in recent years in the USA, while a separate population of pathotypic variants has evolved in Europe. In addition, there has been a world-wide trend towards increasing virulence with Marek's disease virus, and the continuing emergence of antigenic variants of infectious bronchitis virus has caused local difficulties. Thus, if past history is a reliable indicator, we can expect new problems caused by virus diseases to emerge in the future.

The elements of the strategy are as follows: development of an awareness of new diseases, accurate definition of new diseases, determination of their etiology and elucidation of their epidemiology, and finally, development of control measures. These elements are outlined below.

AWARENESS

Fortunately, given the pre-eminence of a comparatively small number of primary breeding companies world-wide, and the considerable traffic in hatching eggs, live birds, meat products and biologicals, there is a good awareness of international disease trends among poultry veterinarians, and new and/or exotic diseases are usually included in a differential diagnosis. However, this is sometimes reflected in a tendency to assume, whenever unexpected problems occur, that this is due to the importation of a new virus or a new disease.

*Department of Agriculture for Northern Ireland, Veterinary Sciences Division, Stormont, Belfast BT4 3SD, Northern Ireland.

Consequently this may result in a failure to properly investigate other more mundane explanations, such as failures in vaccination. There is now also a growing realisation that in the future it will be important to recognise and control subclinical as well as clinical diseases, both from an economic and a welfare viewpoint. For example, it has recently been shown that subclinical IBD and subclinical chicken anemia virus infections are associated with substantial economic losses (McIlroy et al., 1989; McNulty et al., 1991).

DEFINITION

In order that subsequent investigations can progress to a satisfactory conclusion, it is important that new diseases or new forms of endemic diseases should be properly defined in terms of their clinical and pathological features. For new diseases a description based on presenting clinical and gross pathological features is unlikely to be sufficiently precise to be useful. For example, runting stunting syndrome (RSS) has been diagnosed virtually world-wide on the basis of the appearance of runted and stunted broiler chickens with retarded feathering. A plethora of other, inconsistently appearing, signs and lesions has been described, some of which have been regular features in some geographical areas but not in others (McNulty and McFerran, 1993). Given the variety in descriptions of RSS, it is not clear whether we are dealing with:

(a) one universal syndrome of poor growth and retarded feathering, accompanied by a variety of other signs and lesions, perhaps induced by generalised immunosuppression and caused by local secondary agents; or

(b) a number of different syndromes.

This uncertainty regarding the nature of the disease has undermined attempts to determine its etiology and to investigate its epidemiology. If possible, a more restrictive definition should be used when naming new diseases/syndromes. For example, Goodwin et al. (1993) have suggested that RSS should be diagnosed when sicknesses attributable to small intestinal pathophysiological deficits cannot be linked to known nutritional deficiencies or pathogens, and unique small intestinal microscopic lesions are found that contain virus. The nature of the associated virus can then be used to further classify the condition as e.g. reovirus associated enteritis, enterovirus associated enteritis etc.

Where a particular etiologic agent has been associated with a new disease, attempts to determine its presence or absence may be of use in identifying outbreaks of disease in other locations.

ETIOLOGY

When faced with a new disease in the field, certain epidemiological features may indicate whether it is infectious or not, e.g. association with specific breeder flocks, persistence on sites, evidence of spread through direct and indirect contact etc. Confirmation will depend on isolation of the etiologic agent and experimental reproduction of the disease. The failure to identify the etiological agent in some of the new diseases listed in the introduction, coupled with the recognition of a number of new viruses that are difficult or impossible to grow in commonly used in vitro systems (reviewed by McNulty, 1993), underlines the limitations of current diagnostic methods.

In a dual attempt to demonstrate transmissibility and to isolate the causative agent, investigators have experimentally inoculated birds with extracts of organs obtained from field cases of new diseases. In this situation the nature of experimental subject, i.e. breed affected in the field or specific pathogen free (SPF), its age and the route of exposure are of crucial importance. For example, the effects of a putative etiologic agent of RSS on growth are much more difficult to assess in slowly growing SPF chickens than in broilers; conversely there may be a question regarding the susceptibility of broilers because they possess a wide spectrum of maternally derived antibodies. Similarly, although many adenoviruses will produce an 'inclusion body' hepatitis when inoculated parenterally into day-old chicks, they are harmless when given orally to 3-4 week old chicks (most adenovirus infections are acquired horizontally from this age onwards) (M.S. McNulty, unpublished observations). Thus their role as etiologic agents of inclusion body hepatitis in the field is questionable.

While the isolation of a virus from a diseased organ does not necessarily imply cause and effect, the failure to fulfil Koch's postulates experimentally with candidate etiologic agents does not necessarily exclude them as primary causes of disease either. Failure of a genuine etiologic agent to experimentally reproduce the full spectrum of disease seen in the field may be due to absence of predisposing factors in the experimental situation, i.e. stress, management factors, genetics, appropriate secondary agents etc (Kouwenhoven, 1993) or to the logistical difficulty of reproducing a disease with comparatively low morbidity in a limited number of experimentally infected birds.

In most laboratories, isolation of a virus in vitro is dependant upon the ability of the virus to cause a cytopathic effect in cell cultures or a lethal effect in chick embryos. However, not all viruses are cytopathic or embryo lethal. The sensitivity of in vitro virus isolation systems is greatly increased if detection of viral antigen is used as the marker of viral growth rather than ability to produce cytopathology. The easiest and more reliable way to detect viral antigens is by immunofluorescent staining of acetone-fixed cell culture preparations or cryostat sections of appropriate organs or tissues. Some laboratories use immunoperoxidase techniques instead. The use of direct immunofluorescence using pooled sera from birds experimentally inoculated with field material in diagnostic investigations of new diseases may result in detection of unsuspected or new viruses. For example, this approach enabled us to detect an enterovirus-like virus in the intestinal contents of 1-7 day old broilers with RSS. While it is now recognised that many of the 'new' avian enterovirus-like viruses are difficult to grow in cell cultures, attempts to isolate this virus directly were further complicated by the presence of a reovirus, which rapidly outgrew the entero-like virus in all in vitro systems available (McNulty et al., 1984).

The development of monoclonal antibody-based typing methods for discriminating between different isolates of the same virus represents a great advance over conventional pathotyping and polyclonal antiserum-based serotyping techniques. These have been particularly useful in identification of new IBD virus serotypes in the USA (Snyder, 1990) and in diagnosing outbreaks of Newcastle disease in domestic poultry caused by pigeon PMV-1 (Alexander et al., 1985; 1987).

In recent years, virus diagnostic techniques based on detection of viral nucleic acids have been developed. Some of these, e.g. polymerase chain reaction (PCR) amplification of viral nucleic acid sequences have potentially very high sensitivity and specificity and are very much in vogue. However, with most acute virus infections, viral antigen is present in large amounts in infected tissues/organs and can be detected more rapidly, cheaply and easily by immunofluorescence than nucleic acids can be detected by PCR. PCR is most useful if:

(a) the target nucleic acid to be amplified contains sequences which reveal important epidemiological information about the virus in question (e.g. pathotype, serotype or serogroup) (Cavanagh, 1993; McNulty, 1993);

(b) the diagnostic investigation is started some time after the appearance of disease so that only small amounts of virus may be present; or

(c) if latent virus is being sought.

EPIDEMIOLOGY

Unless the clinical signs and pathological lesions of a virus disease are pathognomonic, and unless infection always results in disease, it is essential that diagnostic tests for detecting the virus and/or its antibody are developed before the epidemiology of the disease can be elucidated. Tests for viral antibodies, particularly those such as ELISAs that are comparatively easy to perform and can be carried out in large numbers, are especially useful. They can be used to determine the prevalence of infection, the duration of time the virus has been in a particular location (assuming historical sera are available for testing), whether subclinical infections occur, the commonest age at exposure etc. Testing of SPF flocks will allow an assessment of the likelihood of contamination of poultry vaccines.

Viruses that spread in breeder flocks around peak egg production are likely to be vertically transmitted in the egg. However, where egg transmission occurs, it is usually at a low frequency, i.e. less than 5% embryos infected. Horizontal transmission depends on when, how, and how easily infection is subsequently spread. There may be an inverse age resistance, a developing age resistance or all ages may be equally susceptible. Infections that are spread via the respiratory tract tend to spread faster than those spread by faecal-oral contact. Some viruses have a lower infectious dose$_{50}$ (ID50) for birds than others - viruses with a low ID_{50} will spread faster than those with a high ID_{50}. The duration of virus shedding and titres of virus shed are important factors in the consideration of control measures. Virus that are excreted in high titres over a prolonged period of time are much more difficult to eradicate than those with short periods of excretion. These aspects of the epidemiology of a virus can be assessed by experimental infections and also by analysis of field outbreaks of disease.

Similarly, other important factors such as the resistance of the virus to standard disinfection/fumigation procedures, the ability to infect other avian species and possible vectors can be investigated. It is more difficult to determine whether latency occurs; attempts to reactivate virus by high doses of immunosuppressant drugs and to detect latent genomes by PCR are possible approaches.

CONTROL

The control strategy to be adopted will be dictated by the epidemiological findings. Table 1 lists those epidemiological factors that would favour control of a new virus disease by eradication, i.e. slaughter of diseased flocks. In practice, however, diseases have been eradicated in the absence of many of the factors listed in Table 1.

Table 1: Epidemiological factors favouring control by slaughter of diseased flocks[a]

Pathognomonic signs/lesions
Reliable diagnostics available
Low prevalence
Significant economic impact
No subclinical infections
Short period of virus excretion
Faecal-oral, not respiratory spread
High ID_{50} of causative virus
Horizontal transmission only
No vectors/alternative hosts
No latency
Susceptible to standard disinfection/fumigation methods
If vaccine used, serology can distinguish between vaccinal antibodies and field exposure.

[a]In general, factors are listed in decreasing order of importance.

If a new disease can be eradicated cheaply and comparatively easily, eradication is obviously the best means of control.

In practice however, most virus diseases of poultry are controlled by vaccination. Commercial vaccines are normally either naturally occurring or laboratory attenuated live vaccines or inactivated adjuvanted vaccines. In general live vaccines stimulate good but transitory local mucosal immune responses, whereas inactivated vaccines stimulate good humoral antibody responses. Priming of breeder flocks with live vaccine followed by use of inactivated vaccine is used to produce high levels of maternally derived antibodies that may protect young chicks against early viral challenge. Vaccination regimes in different countries differ depending on the known and perceived risks.

The use of recombinant DNA technology offers the prospect of developing new vaccines against the classical virus diseases and those new diseases caused by viruses that are difficult to grow in laboratory systems or have not yet been attenuated. This might involve insertion and expression of the appropriate viral genes in a suitable vector system, e.g. turkey herpesvirus or fowl pox virus, or development of subunit adjuvanted vaccines through expression of appropriate viral genes in prokaryotic or eukaryotic expression systems. The future use of recombinant vaccines will be determined by their price and their efficacy.

Precise identification of the etiologic agent is not necessarily a pre-requisite for development of effective vaccines. In the past, inoculation with vaccines based on formalised diseased tissues has stimulated immune responses which were sufficient to prevent the development of clinical signs following field exposure. Although the etiologic agent of hydropericardium syndrome has not yet been identified, a formalised vaccine prepared from livers from affected birds has given encouraging results in field trials, even when used in the face of a disease outbreak (Afzal and Ahmad, 1990).

REFERENCES

Afzal, M. and Ahmad, I. (1990). Efficacy of an inactivated vaccine against hydropericardium syndrome in broilers. Vet. Rec. 126, 59-60.

Alexander, D.J., Wilson, G.W.C., Russell, P.H., Lister, S.A. and Parsons, G. (1985). Newcastle disease outbreaks in fowl in Great Britain during 1984. Vet. Rec. 117, 429-434.

Alexander, D.J., Manvell, R.J., Kemp, P.A., Parsons, G., Collins, M.S., Brockman, S., Russell, P.H. and Lister, S.A. (1987). Use of monoclonal antibodies in the characterisation of avian paramyxovirus type 1 (Newcastle disease virus) isolates submitted to an international reference laboratory. Avian Pathol. 16, 553-565.

Cavanagh, D. (1993). Advances in avian diagnostic technology. Proc. Xth International Congress of the World Vet. Poult. Assoc., pp. 57-70.

Fournier, D. and Gaudry, D. (1994). Recent discoveries on waterfowl pathology: a new parvovirus of Muscovy ducks in France. In 'New and Evolving Diseases of Poultry', Eds. M.S. McNulty and J.B. McFerran, in press.

Goodwin, M.A., Davis, J.F., McNulty, M.S., Brown, J. and Player, E.C. (1993). Enteritis (so-called runting stunting syndrome) in Georgia broiler chicks. Avian Dis. 37, 451-458.

Kouwenhoven, B. (1993). Environment, husbandry, genetic and nutritional interactions in infectious diseases in poultry. Proc. Xth International Congress of the World Vet. Poult. Assoc., pp. 113-126.

McIlroy, S.G., Goodall, E.A., and McCracken, R.M. (1989). Economic effects of subclinical infectious bursal disease on broiler production. Avian Pathol. 18, 465-480.

McNulty, M.S., Allan G.M., Connor, T.J., McFerran, J.B. and McCracken, R.M. (1984). An entero-like virus associated with the runting stunting syndrome. Avian Pathol. 13, 429-439.

McNulty, M.S. and McFerran, J.B. (1993). The runting stunting syndrome - general assessment. In 'Virus Infections of Birds'. Eds. J.B. McFerran and M.S. McNulty, Elsevier, Amsterdam, pp. 519-529.

McNulty, M.S. (1993). Recurrent and emerging diseases. Proc. Xth International Congress of the World Vet. Poult. Assoc., pp. 3-17.

McNulty, M.S., McIlroy, S.G., Bruce, D.W. and Todd, D. (1991). Economic effects of subclinical chicken anemia agent infection in broiler chickens. Avian Dis. 35, 263-268.

Snyder, D.B. (1990). Changes in the field status of infectious bursal disease virus. Avian Pathol. 19, 419-423.

DECISION SUPPORT SYSTEMS

CHESS: A DECISION SUPPORT SYSTEM TO ANALYZE INDIVIDUAL SOW-HERD PERFORMANCE

RUUD B.M. HUIRNE and AALT A. DIJKHUIZEN*

To support farmers in managing their herds, the computer system CHESS has been developed. CHESS is a personal computer system, which analyses records of individual swine breeding herds within an economic framework. The system determines strengths and weaknesses in the management of the pig enterprise. CHESS consists of both one decision support system and three expert systems, designed in a modular manner. The decision support system identifies and assesses the importance of relevant deviations between performance and standards. Its output is used in the expert systems that try to find the strengths and weaknesses by combining and evaluating the previously identified deviations. Moreover, CHESS has been validated by method of a field test and the results obtained are presented.

INTRODUCTION

Modern swine breeding is generally characterized by extended herd sizes and narrowed income margins. In the Netherlands for instance, the average number of sows per farm has increased from about 20 in the early 1970s to over 90 by the mid 1980s. In addition to changes in scale, income margin per sow, defined as net return on labour and management as a percentage of gross returns, decreased considerably from approximately 30% to 20% over the same time-period (L.E.I.-C.B.S., 1977, 1989). Thus minor differences in productive performance have an increasing impact on economic results.

It is, therefore, important that farm managers are aware of the strong and weak elements in their farm management. The technique of individual farm analysis can be used to trace such strong and weak elements. The technical and economic records of individual farms are analyzed and signals for the future are provided by highlighting current strengths to be exploited, and weaknesses to be eliminated or improved. Individual farm analysis may include the following three types of analysis (Huirne *et al.*, 1992): (1) trend analysis, comparing actual herd performance with predictions based on a herd's historical data, (2) comparative analysis, comparing actual herd performance with average performance of similar herds, and (3) comparative trend analysis, comparing the historical development of herd performance with the development of performance of similar herds. Each type of analysis involves the following four interrelated stages (Huirne *et al.*, 1992): (1) tracing deviations, (2) weighting deviations, (3) further analysis of deviations, and (4) evaluation of individual farm performance. The technique of individual farm analysis is a general one, and can basically be used for analyzing every type of agricultural enterprise.

---

* Department of Farm Management, Wageningen Agricultural University, Hollandseweg 1, NL-6706 KN Wageningen, The Netherlands

Theoretically, individual farm analysis can be performed manually. However, this is tedious and time consuming and, therefore, it would be more efficient to build the analysis into a computer model. Such a model works fast and can be used by different people, including those who lack the skills required to perform individual farm analysis manually. Because of the declining price-performance ratio of personal computers, computerized analysis is becoming an interesting opportunity for farms (Berg, 1985; Huirne, 1990).

In this paper a system is presented, named CHESS (Computerized Herd Evaluation System for Sows), which uses the technique of individual farm analysis. The system uses records of individual farms and of other (groups of) farms. As a supporting technique for the farm manager, it can be used for early tracing of problems and for determining the maximum amount that could be spent in exploiting or improving farm performance. CHESS has the following features: it (1) has the ability to interface with both external simulation and optimization models for data exchange, and with management information systems for automated data input, (2) provides a basis for the three types of individual farm analysis, (3) is able to handle data from different time-intervals, and (4) is user friendly and suitable for use in the field.

In this paper the four stages of individual farm analysis will be described. Special attention will be given to the integration of the two major sub-systems of CHESS: the decision support systems (DSS) for carrying out the first two stages and the first part of stage 3, and the expert systems (ES) for carrying out the second part of stage 3 and the last stage. Moreover, the results obtained and the outcome of the validation procedure of the system will be presented. Finally, the potential use of the system for further research and application will be discussed.

TRACING DEVIATIONS

Tracing deviations involves three major aspects: (1) measuring farm performance, (2) establishing standards, and (3) comparing farm performance with standards.

An important issue in the measurement of farm performance is data reliability. To be reliable, data must be accurate and consistent. Quarterly technical and economic data of the pig producing enterprise of an individual farm are used for performance monitoring. These data are provided by an information system commonly used on Dutch farms.

The second aspect of tracing deviations concerns the establishment of performance standards. Because satisfactory values of performance varies by type of farm, a single set of standards cannot be provided for all farms (Kay, 1986). CHESS uses three types of standards. The first type concerns the internal standards. Historical farm data with a time-step of three months during the three previous years are analyzed. However, time-step and number of previous years can easily be adjusted by the user of CHESS. Key-issue in this approach is a prediction for the actual time-period (extrapolation) of farm performance, based on historical data. The predictions are then considered as the internal standards. The second and third type of standards concern external standards. Average performance values of similar herds and the trends during the previous three years of these herds are used as standards in CHESS.

During the third aspect of tracing deviations, CHESS compares farm performance with standards. Depending upon the standards used, three types of comparisons are carried out. Because of the many uncertainties in agricultural production, deviations between performance and standards always exist. Questions concerning the relevance of deviations will be answered in the next paragraphs.

WEIGHTING DEVIATIONS

Economic importance

The second stage of individual farm analysis firstly involves the economic weighting of traced performance deviations. Deviations between actual performance and standards will differ and the economic importance of one unit of deviation will vary between variables, depending on their impact on total economic farm performance. Thus the economic importance of deviations differs between farms and should be calculated for each farm separately. Because the relationships between deviations and economic importance may be non-linear for some variables, CHESS calculates the economic importance not per unit deviation but for the actual magnitude of deviation.

As stated above, all deviations are initially assessed in their original dimensions. By calculating the economic importance of deviations, all deviations are converted to the same units and, therefore, comparisons can be made. Because information systems used on swine breeding farms are usually restricted to the individual pig producing enterprise, the most aggregated variable in CHESS is the gross returns minus feed costs per sow per year. This figure counts for all enterprise returns and for the major variable costs, being feed costs of sows and piglets. Fixed costs are not taken into account in this enterprise approach.

The economic importance of deviations is calculated as follows (Huirne *et al.*, 1992). First, performance variables of the sow herd to be analyzed result in a certain value for gross returns minus feed costs per sow per year. Then, each performance variable is consecutively replaced by the corresponding standard, or in other words, the deviations are consecutively added to performance variables, which results in a new value for gross returns minus feed costs per sow per year. The economic importance of a deviation equals the difference between the new and the original value of gross returns minus feed costs per sow per year. If all performance variables have the same value as the standards than there are no deviations and the economic importance of all variables is 0 (zero).

Statistical importance

As a measure of statistical importance, CHESS relates the traced deviation of a variable j (TD_j) to its standard deviation (SD_j). The statistical importance of a deviation increases if the ratio between traced deviation and standard deviation increases. In mathematical terms:

$$SI_j = TD_j / SD_j \qquad (1)$$

where:

SI_j = statistical importance of a deviation in performance variable j
TD_j = traced deviation of a performance variable j
SD_j = standard deviation of a performance variable j.

Standard deviations must be obtained for each of the three types of analysis. Standard deviations for trend analysis are calculated in CHESS as the square root of estimated residual variance of the linear trend model used for obtaining the predictions. For comparative analysis, standard deviations of the group of similar farms are regularly made available in the Netherlands by the National Extension Service (Baltussen *et al.*, 1988). For comparative trend analysis, the standard deviations required to determine statistical importance of deviations are also obtained from external sources.

Relevance of a deviation

In determining the relevance of a deviation, CHESS takes into account both its economic and statistical importance. The relevance of a deviation is calculated by multiplying the economic importance with the absolute value of the statistical importance of a deviation in performance variable j. In formula:

$$RD_j = EI_j * |SI_j| \qquad (2)$$

where:

RD_j = relevance of a deviation in performance variable j
EI_j = calculated economic importance of a deviation in performance variable j (in Dfl.)
SI_j = calculated statistical importance of a deviation in performance variable j.

The absolute value in the formula is used only to avoid changes in sign in the economic importance of a deviation. Thus, economic importance and relevance of a deviation always have the same sign.

As an illustration, an example is given in Table 1.

Table 1. Calculation of the relevance of deviations for some variables (abbreviations: see text)

Variable j	AV_j	SV_j	TD_j	SD_j	$\|SI_j\|$	EI_j	RD_j
1. litters/sow/year	2.01	2.15	-0.14	0.10	1.40	-99	-139
2. pigs born alive/litter	10.80	10.67	0.13	0.50	0.26	17	4
3. % pig mortality	18.00	15.21	2.79	4.40	0.63	-46	-29
4. feeder pigs sold/litter	8.86	9.05	-0.19	0.60	0.32	-29	-9
5. feeder pigs sold/sow/year	17.80	19.45	-1.65	2.00	0.83	-149	-123
6. pig feed per pig (kg)	25.00	29.04	-4.04	2.40	1.68	60	100
7. sow feed/sow/year (kg)	1070.15	1107.78	-37.63	64.70	0.58	19	11

With respect to the first variable (j = 1), actual value (AV_1) of litters per sow per year is 2.01, and standard value (SV_1) is 2.15. So, the traced deviation (TD_1) equals -0.14. With standard deviation (SD_1) being 0.10, the absolute value of the statistical importance is 1.40. The relevance of the deviation (RD_1) can then be determined (-139) by multiplying the absolute value of statistical importance (SI_1) by Dfl. -99, the calculated economic importance of the deviation (EI_1). Using this formula, all deviations are on the same scale and easily compared.

FURTHER ANALYSIS OF DEVIATIONS

The third stage of individual farm analysis is a further analysis of deviations. In determining deviations that must be subject to further analysis, all deviations are screened for relevance. As discussed before, deviations between performance and standards always exist. The question is at what level of deviation do they become relevant. For this purpose CHESS uses the so-called relevance diagram (Fig. 1).

The relevance diagram helps to determine important levels of deviation. Relevant deviations may be intolerable if they have a negative economic importance (weaknesses) or be desirable if they have a positive economic importance (strengths). The diagram is based on the principle of double relevance. If the relevance of a deviation varies around zero (stage 0), it is presumed that the deviation is irrelevant, and no further analysis is needed. If the deviation falls into stage 1, it may be relevant and a previous time-period is checked and the deviation is defined as relevant if it is the result of a slow change in performance. In case of stage 2, the deviation is considered to be relevant, and subject to further analysis. The diagram is symmetrical around zero, treating positive relevance of deviations in the same way as negative relevance. The choice of (user defined) boundaries, determines the level of analysis. If narrow boundaries are chosen, a greater number of differences will be relevant. If wide boundaries are chosen, the converse is true.

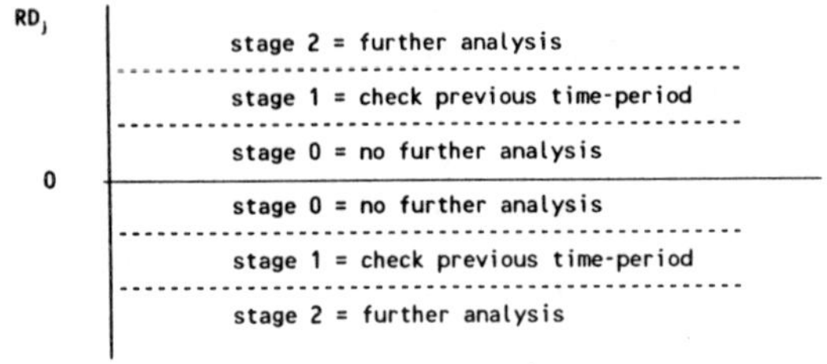

Fig. 1. The relevance diagram used in CHESS (RD_j = Relevance of a Deviation in performance variable j)

The relevance diagram in its present form is used for all deviations within trend analysis and comparative analysis. For comparative trend analysis it is not valid to use stage 1 of the relevance diagram. Therefore, stage 1 is eliminated and stage 2 covers the range of relevances formerly covered by stages 1 and 2.

Performance deviations that are relevant are subject to further analysis. In practice, analysis of deviations is not worthwhile unless the factors that caused them are identified (Anthony and Dearden, 1980). Therefore, further analysis of deviations requires the combination of deviations to find common causes. First, deviations should be divided into those that are to be controlled by an individual farm manager and those that are not. Because results of the analysis should be interpreted and used as a guide for management decisions, further analysis is performed only on those deviations that are under manager control. To find causes, deviations should be related to each other to see to what extent relevant deviations are associated. This is a difficult process, for which years of special training and experience are normally required.

In finding causes it may be valuable to find out that some deviations are relevant and others are not. So, information both on relevance and irrelevance of deviations can be very important. However, further analysis is started on the basis of relevant deviations. This is commonly called management by exception (Anthony, 1970; Castle *et al.*, 1987). The exceptions or relevant deviations between performance and standards are symptoms of strong and weak elements. These symptoms are then analyzed to pinpoint the cause of these elements. Management's attention is thus focused on a relatively small number of relevant deviations.

EVALUATION OF INDIVIDUAL FARM PERFORMANCE

During the last stage of individual farm analysis, deviations and causal factors are evaluated by CHESS. To obtain a good indication of individual farm performance, causes of relevant deviations should be considered together with the initial farm data, established standards, and calculated economic importance of deviations. Evaluating farm performance is a very difficult process. There is also a close relationship between the method of evaluation and the method of finding causes of performance deviations. CHESS uses expertise from human experts (rules of thump and heuristics) in these two stages (evaluation and (second part of) further analysis). For this reason, the activities mentioned above are carried out by the expert systems of CHESS. The global structure of such an expert system is outlined in Fig. 2. The global structure includes the following areas of special attention: nutrition, health care, reproduction, housing, input/output of animals, and prices. These areas may be divided further into some sub-areas.

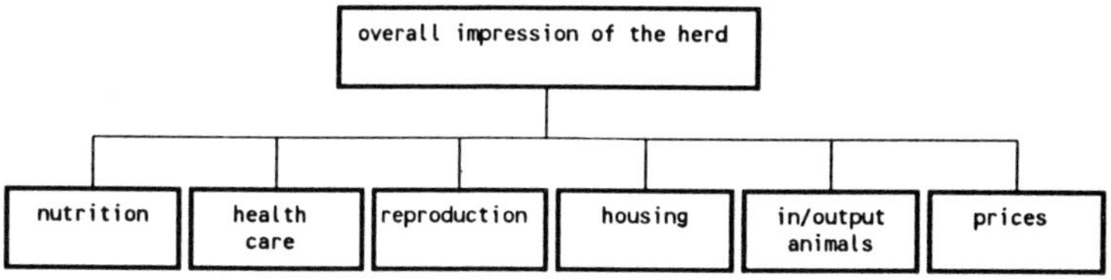

Fig. 2. Global structure of the expert systems of CHESS

By means of illustration, the following production rule, which is derived from human expertise and used in a CHESS expert system, is presented.

RULE 10

IF	Percent remating of sows is high OR Interval first mating-conception of sows is high
AND	Number of pigs total born per litter is low
THEN	There is a suggestive evidence (0.60) that the mating moment of the sows is wrong

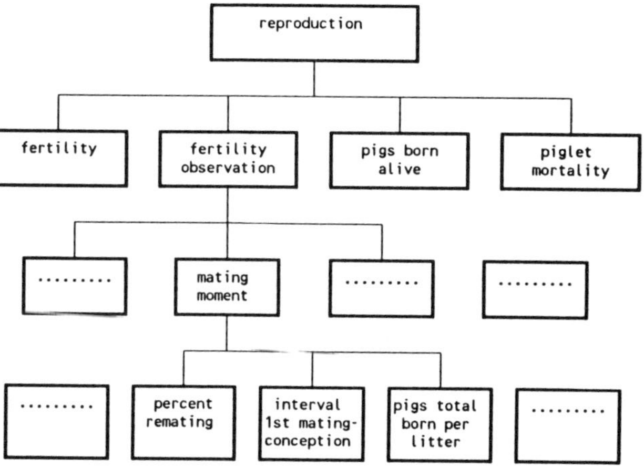

Fig. 3. Structure of the reproduction area in CHESS

RULE 10 is one of the rules in the reproduction area. Within the reproduction area it belongs to the fertility observation sub-area. In Fig. 3, RULE 10 is implemented in the structure of the reproduction area.

Once strengths and weaknesses have been identified, a farm manager may choose an appropriate course of action for dealing with these elements.

VALIDATION OF THE COMPUTER SYSTEM CHESS

General concepts of validation

Validation is an important stage in developing computerized systems, to be described as comparing the computer system with the real world (Gilchrist, 1984). Measurement of the validity of any system, however, is a difficult issue. This is especially so when ES are considered where, as described above, symbolic problem solving techniques and heuristics are used to produce conclusions (Harrison, 1991). This may partially explain why no validation methods for ES could be found in literature.

In validating any system, attention should be focused on that part of the real world which is represented (McCarl, 1984; Harrison, 1991). It is not necessary to reflect the real world perfectly, but it is essential to abstract reality such that it is adequate for the system's anticipated use. The process of validation in this paper is divided into "internal" and "external" validation (Taylor, 1983; Huirne *et al.*, 1991). Internal validation concerns ensuring that the right answer, decision or recommendation is provided by the correct method, and that each equation or part of the system has a logical basis, uses correct parameters and is correctly written. A system can also be validated externally by comparing its performance against the performance of the real world, in which the system is considered as a "black box". Because systems are usually unable to reproduce or predict the entire real environment, external validity must conclude whether the use of the system is appropriate for the observed and expected errors. This may include a sensitivity analysis in which the values of the parameters used in the system are systematically varied over some range of interest to determine whether and how the solution or recommendation changes (Anderson, 1974; Dent and Blackie, 1979).

Validation of CHESS

After internal validation, which did not result in "hard" quantitative facts, CHESS was validated externally. Because of the qualitative character of the output obtained, CHESS could not be validated using pure statistical methods. So, external validation of CHESS was restricted to a non-statistical method i.e. carrying out a field test. The field test of CHESS should indicate the strong and weak elements in the performance of the system compared to the performance of experts. Ten herds were randomly selected from two major swine breeding regions in the Netherlands. The field test was performed as follows. The experts made an individual farm analysis of the ten herds, using the farm data provided by their information system and other information available. To facilitate comparison, pre-defined areas of special attention should be considered. The experts were asked to analyze each herd using their usual protocol and taking the same amount of time. The experts were then requested to put certainty factors (CF) or probability weightings on their detected strong and weak elements in the farm management. After the ten farm were analyzed by the experts, they were analyzed by CHESS. Finally, the results of the expert analyses were compared with the results of CHESS.

The conclusions of both the experts and CHESS were connected with CF. To evaluate the performances, the CF of the conclusions were divided into three classes. Conclusions CF which equaled 0 (zero) were placed in class A, CF values between 0.01 and 0.34 in class B, and CF values greater than 0.35 in class C. The agreement between the results of CHESS and experts is summarized in Table 2.

The percent test agreement (PTA) between CHESS and the experts, defined as percent CF values classified into the same classes (A, B and C), can be calculated using Table 2. The PTA turned out to be 60% ((398+84+35)/840). In the field CHESS should be used as a system for early detecting of problems or opportunities and it is, therefore, important that it does not overlook the early stages of such changes. Table 2 provides also a basis for calculating the occurrence of such errors. CHESS may be considered to have overlooked strengths or weakness if the CF given by the system fell into class A while the corresponding CF given by the experts fell into the classes B or C. The percent mis-classification errors turned out to be 4% ((35+1)/ 840). So, the knowledge of the experts has successfully been incorporated into the computerized system CHESS.

Table 2. The results of CHESS compared to the results of the experts

		RESULTS OF EXPERTS			
	CLASS*	A	B	C	TOTAL
	A	398**	35	1	434
RESULTS OF	B	139	84	15	238
CHESS	C	83	60	25	168
	TOTAL	620	179	41	840

*class A: CF = 0, class B: 0.01 ≤ CF ≤ 0.34, class C: CF ≥ 0.35
**numbers refer to the total number of conclusions involved

DISCUSSION AND OUTLOOK

CHESS can be divided into two major parts: the DSS-part and ES-part. In the DSS-part, the problems of interest (included in the first two stages and the first part of stage 3 of individual farm analysis) are fairly well structured, and DSS techniques are used to solve them. On the other hand, in the ES-part, the problems of interest (included in stage 3 (second part) and stage 4 of individual farm analysis) are relatively poorly structured and expert practitioners provide a powerful source of successful procedures for problem solving. These procedures have the additional advantage that they are fitted to the information handling capabilities of human problem solvers (Johnson, 1983). CHESS integrates DSS and ES to combine their advantages for a more valuable synergetic system. Results of the quantitative DSS analysis of individual farm performance are used as ES input. The ES combines and evaluates these results to find strong and weak elements in farm management and organization.

An important issue in determining the boundaries in the relevance diagram is that a small deviation between farm performance and a standard can be the start of a sizable and permanent deviation over future periods, while in other cases a small deviation may be a coincidence and of short term duration. It is desirable to detect the first situation at an early stage so that further analysis and corrective actions can be taken rapidly. In the second situation no further analysis is required, and inappropriate responses should be avoided. Relevant deviations may be either those with a negative economic importance (weaknesses or problems) or positive economic importance (strengths). Corrective actions may be either to improve weaknesses or to exploit strengths using knowledge on factors that caused them.

CHESS includes three types of analysis. This provides for the detection of the most important strengths and weaknesses in the management of a farm. However, conflicting results may be obtained between each type of analysis. For instance, reproduction may be indicated a strong point in trend analysis, but a problem in comparative analysis. It is difficult to cope with this problem. Therefore, CHESS presents the results of each type of analysis separately, giving farm managers the opportunity to choose the type they consider the most appropriate.

It is important to measure the quality of output of CHESS. Since CHESS contains three ES, which use symbolic problem solving techniques and heuristics to draw conclusions, validation is also difficult. The soundness of relationships in an ES can usually be examined against (biological) logic and published scientific research. The heuristics built into an ES are less readily validated. However, as described before, a field test can be used to gain insight into the strong and weak elements of a computer system. The promising validation results obtained for CHESS suggest that it has a potential practical application.

Using CHESS for analyzing the performance of individual sow herds, the major strong and weak elements in management are traced, and their economic impact is calculated. Where serious problems (weak elements) are found by CHESS, a more detailed analysis in depth of such problems could be necessary. Therefore, other systems must be developed for further analysis of these smaller areas, using more - and more detailed - farm data on such area. Potential areas are nutrition (for analysis of feeding-scheme for example), health care (for analysis of vaccination-program) and reproduction (for analysis of the replacement policy). If these systems become available and can be integrated into CHESS, a powerful and useful system will be obtained for detailed analysis of the whole herd, and, if necessary, a detailed analysis in depth of certain (strong or weak) elements within the herd. Further research is going on to provide these systems.

REFERENCES

Anderson, J.R. (1974). Simulation: methodology and applications in agricultural economics. Review of Marketing and Agricultural Economics 65, 3-55.

Anthony, R.N. (1970). Management accounting: text and cases. Irwin, Homewood, IL.

Anthony, R.N. and Dearden, J. (1980). Management control systems. Irwin, Homewood, IL.

Baltussen, W.H.M., Altena, H., Bakker, C.M., and Van Rijnberk, D. (1988). Results on Dutch swine breeding herds in 1987. Swine Extension Service and Agricultural Economics Research Institute, Rosmalen.

Berg, E. (1985). Microcomputereinsatz im landwirtschaftlichen Betrieb. Berichte über Landwirtschaft 63, 376-389.

Castle, E.N., Becker, M.H. and Nelson, A.G. (1987). Farm business management. The decision-making process. Macmillan, New York.

Dent, J.B. and Blackie, M.J. (1979). Systems simulation in agriculture. Applied Science, London.

Gilchrist, W. (1984). Statistical modelling. Wiley, Chichester.

Harrison, S.R. (1991). Validation of agricultural expert systems. Agricultural Systems 35, 265-285.

Huirne, R.B.M. (1990). Basic concepts of computerized support for farm management decisions. European Review of Agricultural Economics 17, 69-84.

Huirne, R.B.M., Dijkhuizen, A.A. and Backus, G.B.C. (1991). Validation of an integrated decision support and expert system for analysis of individual sow-herd performance. Computers and Electronics in Agriculture 6, 71-86.

Huirne, R.B.M., Dijkhuizen, A.A., Renkema, J.A. and Van Beek, P. (1992). Computerized analysis of individual sow-herd performance. American Journal of Agricultural Economics 74, 388-399.

Johnson, P.E. (1983). What kind of expert should a system be? The Journal of Medicine and Philosophy 8, 77-97.

Kay, R.D. (1986). Farm management. Planning, control, and implementation. McGraw-Hill, New York.

L.E.I.-C.B.S. (1977,1989). Figures of Dutch Agriculture. Agricultural Economics Research Institute and Netherlands Central Bureau of Statistics, The Hague.

McCarl, B.A. (1984). Model validation: an overview with some emphasis on risk models. Review of Marketing and Agricultural Economics 52, 153-173.

Taylor, A.J. (1983). The verification of dynamic simulation models. Journal of Operational Research Society 34, 233-242.

EQUINE EPIDEMIOLOGY

THE DEVELOPMENT OF EQWISE - EQUINE WELFARE INFORMATION SYSTEM / EXPERT

D.J. MELLOR[1] , S.W.J. REID[1], T. IRWIN[2], C.W. REVIE[3], AND G. GETTINBY[2]

EQWISE has been developed as the result of a two year feasibility study commissioned by The Home of Rest for Horses. The objective of the study was to develop powerful integrated knowledge management tools to allow widespread distribution of information relating to equine disease and welfare. In order to achieve this, a multidisciplinary approach was adopted which has led to the formation of The Veterinary Informatics and Health Group, a joint initiative between The Department of Veterinary Medicine, University of Glasgow and The Department of Statistics and Modelling Science, University of Strathclyde. The result has been the harnessing of expertise from the domains of veterinary science, information science and mathematical disease modelling to address the challenges posed by the objective of the study.

There were three separate but related areas of development. First, data generated from all research projects previously funded by The Home of Rest for Horses was committed to electronic format, collated and restructured to allow systematic interrogation of the information. Secondly, a large scale survey of the equine population of Scotland and Northern England was initiated through veterinarians and horse owners in order to identify the population of horses at risk from disease. Thirdly, clinical heuristics were devised to develop an expert system to assist in the diagnosis of coughing in horses.

The three components have been integrated and developed as a PC (Personal Computer) application running in Microsoft Windows. The choice of a Windows / PC combination makes EQWISE both user friendly and available to as many potential users as possible.

CREATION OF AN ELECTRONIC LIBRARY

The collation of archival information supplied by The Home of Rest for Horses has provided the basis of an electronic library containing seven PhD theses, one MSc thesis, a publication

---

[1] Department of Veterinary Medicine, University of Glasgow Veterinary School, Bearsden Road, Glasgow G61 1QH

[2] Department of Statistics and Modelling Science and [3] Department of Information Science, University of Strathclyde, George Street, Glasgow G1 1XW

entitled 'Contributions to Equine Welfare' and other miscellaneous reports. The commitment to electronic format involved the scanning of individual pages of text using optical character recognition software. Photographic plates, tables and illustrations were also scanned to produce electronic images. Structural links were created between related 'nodes' of information so that a user might easily follow a specific theme through any particular document. This type of linking is referred to as hypertext (Nielsen, 1990), (Woodhead, 1991). EQWISE has been built using KnowledgePro Gold© (Knowledge Garden Inc. USA), a high level programming language particularly suited to developing hypertext applications for Windows.

Selecting 'Library' from the menu bar of EQWISE opens a window on the screen listing the documents contained in the electronic library and some summary information concerning the size and subject matter of each document. The user may select any document and open it by clicking the 'Open' button which appears in the contents window. Opening a document brings up a window displaying the structural breakdown of that document (chapter headings which are highlighted in blue indicating a hypertext link to another part of the document). Clicking a chapter heading allows the user to move to another window showing the breakdown of that chapter (subheadings highlighted in the same way as before). Selecting a subheading opens a window containing the relevant section of text. A scrollbar on the right side of the window allows the user to move through the section of text on the screen. Links appear highlighted in the text based on a colour coding: links to other text in blue, links to figures in magenta, links to tables in red and links to references in green. A single mouse click takes the user to the relevant piece of text, or displays the relevant figure, table or reference in a window on the screen. References that are displayed on the screen can be added to a list which can be printed out if required. Two buttons, 'Contents' and 'Back', are located at the top of the text window. Clicking the 'Contents' button allows the user to view the contents page (usually the chapter headings) of the document that is open. Clicking the 'Back' button returns the user to the section of text from which they moved to the present section. A "history trail" can also be displayed in the text window which shows all the sections visited previously.

The electronic library contains a search facility. The user can search for a specific word or string of words in any or all documents contained in the library. On completion of the search the user is presented with a window containing a list of all sections of text where the search term was found. Clicking on any list item will then take the user to that particular section, where every occurrence of the search term is highlighted in the text.

DEMOGRAPHIC CENSUS

A survey was designed to identify the population of horses in Scotland and Northern England at risk from disease. The survey took the form of a mail questionnaire (Dillman, 1978), (Vaillancourt, 1991) and was carried out with the co-operation of veterinarians and horse owners in the area. The survey was implemented in three stages:

1. Survey of Veterinary Practices
2. Population Survey
3. Disease and Welfare Survey

Twenty-five veterinary practices spread throughout Scotland and Northern England were identified and contacted by telephone. All practices agreed to take part in the study, and were asked to complete a questionnaire concerning the quantity and nature of equine work undertaken. Practitioners were also asked to comment on the frequency with which different diseases were diagnosed and to indicate which disease or diseases were the most important in terms of equine welfare. All horse owning clients of the twenty-five practices were mailed a simple questionnaire concerning the number of horses they owned, where and how these animals were kept and the purpose for which they were used. The questionnaire also asked horse owners if they would be prepared to complete a supplementary, more detailed, questionnaire concerning the disease and welfare of their animals. Owners who were prepared to do so were asked to include their name and address so that the supplementary questionnaire could be mailed to them. The data gathered from the Population Survey provided baseline information on the distribution, numbers, management and use of equine animals throughout Scotland and Northern England. A random sample of horse owning respondents from the Population Survey was then taken to be included in the Disease and Welfare Survey.

Twenty-two of the twenty-five veterinary practices completed the questionnaire. Together these practices provided veterinary care for approximately 17,500 horses owned by approximately 8,500 people. On average equine work comprised approximately 20% of the total practice workload, with vaccination, certification and other routine tasks making up approximately 45% of this work. Lameness was considered to be the most significant welfare problem in horses, with laminitis cited most frequently as the cause of this. COPD, endoparasite infection and poor management were also felt to be frequent causes of suffering in horses.

From the Population Survey approximately 35% of horse owners own only one horse, but >50% of horses are kept in groups of 5 or more. Approximately 13% of horses are permanently grazed whereas only 2% are permanently stabled, the remaining 85% spending varying proportions of their time stabled and grazing. The most popular uses of horses are: hacking (18%), breeding (15%), riding and pony club events (14%).

At the time of writing the Disease and Welfare Questionnaire is under development. The results of the Disease and Welfare Survey will be integrated with those summarised here and compared to those from the Survey of Veterinary Practices. A Geographical Information System (GIS) software package (running in Microsoft Windows) will be used to plot the distribution of horses and their diseases throughout Scotland and Northern England and relate these data to environmental factors (Kendall, 1991), (Cadoux-Hudson & Heywood, 1992).

Davies (1983) in a discussion of programmes concluded that disease surveillance consumes vast resources in staff time and thought. The alternative is to have detailed knowledge of populations; their numbers, distribution and age structure and to mount point prevalence surveys, finite longitudinal investigations, case control studies and other exercises that are designed to answer considered questions. The census component of EQWISE will catalogue the demographic characteristics of the UK equine population. The disease prevalence data highlight those areas equine health and welfare in need of further, more detailed research.

THE DEVELOPMENT OF A COUGH CONSULTATION SYSTEM

The EQWISE Cough Consultation System is an expert system (Turban, 1990) which has been developed to assist in the diagnosis of coughing in horses. Eighteen clinical conditions (or condition groupings) that are likely to cause coughing in horses were identified by a panel of veterinary clinicians. Heuristics were defined on the basis of clinical findings which differentiate between these conditions. A series of questions concerning the clinical presentation of an animal or group of animals is posed sequentially to the user by the system. The user responds to each question by clicking the appropriate answer in the 'Questions' box. The answer given then appears in the 'Answers' list box and any conditions that are ruled out on the basis of this answer appear adjacent to it in the 'Rejected Conditions' list box. The consultation proceeds with answers to subsequent questions further reducing the differential list of conditions remaining in the 'Possible Conditions' list box. In the course of a consultation a user can be left with only one condition remaining in the 'Possible Conditions' box, before having answered all the questions posed by the system. Should this occur a message appears on the screen advising that all the questions should be answered as the remaining condition could be rejected by a subsequent answer. When all the conditions are rejected the user is advised to re-examine the animal as the answers given are unlikely to reflect the clinical presentation of an animal suffering solely from a disease of which coughing is the major clinical sign. At the end of a consultation, when all the questions have been answered, (or at any point during a consultation) the user can access reference sections on any of the disease conditions in the system. These sections comprise hypertext subsections and contain information on aetiology, epidemiology, pathogenesis, diagnosis, treatment and prevention of each condition. Hypertext links to radiographs, photomicrographs, endoscopic photographs are included in diagnosis subsections, and links to drugs and their data sheets are included in treatment and prevention sections. It is possible to link from this 'Cough Reference Text' to the electronic library and demographic census components of EQWISE.

DISCUSSION

The completion of the two-year feasibility study has seen the development of a knowledge retrieval system which contains information relevant to equine welfare. The integration of the three parts of the system shows how different types of information can be related as composite units in one interface. This allows a user to perform a more complete interrogation of knowledge contained in the system by providing the opportunity to consider not only a particular topic of interest but also any information related to that topic. Running the system in Microsoft Windows makes it intuitive and easy to use as all functions are implemented by mouse clicks. The user is not required to type any complicated commands which would greatly reduce the speed with which an interrogation of the system could be completed.

The system has potential for development in the areas of veterinary practice, research, undergraduate teaching and as a reference for welfare organisations and research funding bodies. It is perceived that these separate areas will require EQWISE to be developed in a different way for each type of potential end user.

The future development of EQWISE will include an extension of the demographic census to the whole of the UK. GIS technology (Maguire et al., 1991) will be used as a means of representing the distribution of the equine population, its disease and welfare problems and their relation to environmental factors. Such a system has scope as a preventive medical tool by helping to predict patterns of disease spread and highlighting associated environmental features (Morris et al., 1993). Expert system modules will be developed to deal with other major clinical syndromes such as pruritus, lameness, colic, diarrhoea and wasting. In order to do justice to these complicated areas, the use of multimedia will be investigated so that audio and video features can be incorporated into the consultation modules. The large database of biochemical records of equine cases referred to the University of Glasgow Veterinary Hospital will be analysed to relate biochemical abnormalities to clinical and pathological findings. These clinicopathological indices will then be incorporated into the diagnostic support modules of the system along with mathematical disease models under development in The Veterinary Informatics and Health Group.

With rapid advances in veterinary science it is becoming impossible for any individual to remain conversant with all the most recent information in all areas of the subject. Computer systems can never replace clinicians or teachers or researchers: their role is in providing access to large volumes of knowledge structured in such a way as to yield the greatest amount of relevant information with the greatest efficiency. The combination of veterinary clinical expertise and information technology can contribute a great deal to increasing the awareness of animal disease and welfare issues. The end result will be a prioritisation of problem areas in terms of future research funding, leading to a greater understanding of disease and subsequent improvement in animal welfare.

ACKNOWLEDGEMENTS

The authors would like to thank Professor M. Murray and Dr. S. Love (University of Glasgow Veterinary School) and Dr. W. D. Tavernor (The Home of Rest for Horses). This project was funded by The Home of Rest for Horses.

REFERENCES

Cadoux-Hudson, J. and Heywood, D.I. (1992). The Yearbook of the Association for Geographic Information. Taylor & Francis, London, 1992.

Davies, G. (1983). Development of Veterinary Epidemiology. The Veterinary Record, 112, 51-53.

Dillman, D.A., (1978). Mail and Telephone Surveys. John Wiley and Sons Inc., New York, N.Y.

Kendall, R. (1991). Mapping Software - Analyzing a World of Data. PC Magazine, July 1991, 249-275.

Morris, R.S., Sanson, R.L., McKenzie, J.S. and Marsh, W.E. Decision Support Systems in Animal Health. Society for Veterinary Epidemiology and Preventive Medicine, proceedings of a meeting held at the University of Exeter, 31 March - 2 April 1993.

Maguire, D.J., Goodchild, M.F. and Rhind, D.W. (1991). Geographical Information

Systems: Principles and Applications. Harlow, Essex Longman Scientific and Technical.

Nielsen, J. (1990). Hypertext and Hypermedia. Boston, Academic Press, 1990.

Turban, E. (1993). Decision Support and Expert Systems. Third Edition. Collier Macmillan Publishers, London, 1993.

Vaillancourt, J-P., Martineau, G., Morrow, M., Marsh, W., Robinson, A. Construction of Questionnaires and their use in Veterinary Medicine. Society for Veterinary Epidemiology and Preventive Medicine, proceedings of a meeting held at the University of London, 17-19 April 1991.

Woodhead, N. (1991). Hypertext and Hypermedia: theory and applications. Sigma Press, 1991.

PRELIMINARY ANALYSIS OF A MATCHED CASE CONTROL STUDY OF GRASS SICKNESS IN THE UNITED KINGDOM

J.L.N. WOOD[*], D.L.DOXEY[**] AND E.M.MILNE[**]

INTRODUCTION

Grass Sickness, or equine dysautonomia is a disease of horses of unknown aetiology. Disruption of the enteric autonomic nervous systems results in disturbance of intestinal movement. Clinical cases present with colic, difficulties in swallowing and defecating and failure of gastric emptying with subsequent reflux. The severity varies from the most severe, per-acute cases, all of which will rapidly die, to the less severe cases with a slower onset with severe weight loss and a better prognosis.

The disease is characterised histologically by degeneration of neurones in the autonomic ganglia (Obel, 1955; Gilmour, 1975) and a loss of neurones in myenteric plexi (Doxey *et al.*, 1992). The principal histological change in the autonomic ganglia is chromatolysis (Obel, 1955; Gilmour, 1975a); neuronal loss and neuronophagia are also seen.

Previous epidemiological investigations have been carried out in Scotland and have identified factors associated with increased risk of grass sickness. Gilmour and Jolly (1974), in a prospective case control study, showed that horses at particular risk were those at grass aged between two and seven years old, particularly if they had been on the premises for less than two months. Horses grazing on premises where grass sickness had previously been recorded were also at increased risk, particularly if grass sickness had occurred in the previous two years. Horses receiving hay and concentrate were at reduced risk, although those at grass just receiving concentrate were at significantly increased risk when compared to those receiving no supplementary feeding (figures in Gilmour 1975b). Those horses receiving hay alone as a supplementary feed were at equal risk to those receiving no supplementary feed. Doxey *et al* (1991a) also showed an association with age, grazing, recent movement and condition of the horse.

Grass sickness is a seasonal disease, with most cases being observed in early summer (especially May and June) and there has been an anecdotal association between grass sickness and cold dry weather for many years (Pool, 1927; Greig, 1942; Gilmour, 1975b). Doxey *et al.* (1991b) demonstrated a trend towards cool dry weather preceding outbreaks of grass sickness.

---

[*] Department of Infectious Diseases, Animal Health Trust, P.O.Box 5, Newmarket, SUFFOLK CB8 7DW

[**] Department of Veterinary Clinical Studies, Royal (Dick) School of Veterinary Studies, University of Edinburgh, Veterinary Field Station, Easter Bush, Roslin, Midlothian EH25 9RG.

The two major comparative epidemiological studies of grass sickness (Gilmour and Jolly, 1974 and Doxey *et al.*, 1991a) both collected control data at different times to the case data. As many of the factors predisposing towards grass sickness relate to management, both studies have been unable to exclude the possibility of bias due to management changing with season. Moreover, all previous epidemiological studies of grass sickness in the UK have restricted themselves to certain geographic regions. A case control study of cases of grass sickness in the United Kingdom was therefore carried out, with control data collected at the same time as case data to evaluate the role of predisposing factors. The results are intended to improve our ability to prevent the disease and increase our understanding of the likely aetiology.

MATERIALS AND METHODS

The study was based on a user friendly questionnaire which recorded data on horse, premises, weather and management. Each questionnaire recorded information on only one horse. It was designed to be completed by owners, although some were returned by veterinary surgeons. The study was advertised through the Equine Grass Sickness Fund and the media, including local television, radio, magazines and newspapers.

Owners were requested to contact the Animal Health Trust (AHT) or the Grass Sickness Fund if a horse suffered grass sickness. Also, the owners of all cases of grass sickness presented at the Royal (Dick) School of Veterinary Studies were asked to join the study. They were then given or sent a set of three questionnaires and reply paid envelope, with a request to fill in one for the case of grass sickness, another for a healthy horse on the same premises and the third for a healthy horse on another premises. Owners were asked to answer the questions as on the day of clinical onset of grass sickness in the case.

Data Recording and Analysis

Data were entered into Epi-info version 5 (Dean *et al.*, 1990). After 'cleaning', they were then transferred into Egret (1989) for statistical analysis. The basic method of analysis was conditional logistic regression, as required for matched case control studies (Breslow and Day, 1980). Sets were matched on the incident of grass sickness. After univariate analysis, multivariate models were fitted by experimentation and confirmed by forward stepwise regression with an entry level of $\alpha=0.05$.

Some questions related to the premises and others to the weather. As all controls were matched by date and half additionally by premises, no differences were expected between cases and controls on these questions, particularly when considering the controls on the same premises.

Questionnaire

The questions were generally answered by means of ticking the box. The questions (and some others) covered in the preliminary analyses are summarised in Table 1. Other questions not been included due to very low proportions of positive responses from both cases and controls.

Table 1. Summary of some of questions included in grass sickness questionnaire.

To what type of horse does this questionnaire apply?	i) Grass sickness ii) Well and on same premises iii) Well and on another premises	Bodily Condition	i) Fat ii) Good iii) Thin
Height	(hands)	Age	(years or months)
Type of Grazing (if outdoors at all)	i) Hill/Moor ii) Permanent Grass iii) Ley seeded w/i 4 yr iv) Water Meadow v) Other	Sex/Breeding Status	i) Gelding ii) Stallion/Colt iii) Mare iv) Pregnant Mare
Present Management	i) Entirely Outdoors ii) Part Outdoors/Part Stabled iii) Entirely Stabled	Move of Pasture w/i 6 months	i) No ii) Yes & when moved
Previous Management	i) Entirely Outdoors ii) Part Outdoors/Part Stabled iii) Entirely Stabled iv) Not moved	Supplementary Feed	i) Hay or not & amount ii) Silage or not & amount iii) Cut grass or not & amount iv) Milled Concentrate or not & amount v) Corn/Any Grain or not & amount
Worming History	i) Never been wormed ii) Wormed annually iii) Every six months iv) Every 2 months v) More than twice monthly	Vaccination against tetanus	i) No ii) Yes and date
Time on Premises	(number of weeks or months)	Previous GS on Premises	i) Yes ii) No
Time of Previous Grass Sickness	i) Yes & When ii) Yes but not sure of date iii) Never before	Was previous case grazing same field as your horse	i) Yes ii) No
Was horse on premises at time of previous gs	i) Yes ii) No	Was horse in contact of previous case	i) Yes ii) No
Total no. horses on premises	(Number)	Total number in same field	number & give approx. field size
Preceding Weather Conditions	i) Mostly Dry ii) Mostly Showery iii) Mostly Wet	Preceding Weather Conditions	i) Hot (17°C or more) ii) Warm (12-16°C) iii) Cool (11°C or less)
Are you aware of rabbits grazing premises?	i) No ii) Yes and appeared well iii) Yes and sick or behaving abnormally.	Are you aware of hares grazing premises?	i) No ii) Yes and appeared well iii) Yes and sick or behaving abnormally.
Method of Diagnosis (cases only)	i) On Clinical Signs ii) After post-mortem iii) After PM with histology	Date of Death (cases only)	(date)

RESULTS.

Return rates: 215 questionnaires were sent out to owners of horses with grass sickness or their veterinary surgeons. 97 completed questionnaires were received, although 16 returned data only on the case without any control data. The response rate is summarised in Table 2. Due to the method of analysis, all sets that only included case data were automatically excluded. There were thus 81 matched sets usable in the analysis.

Table 2. Questionnaire Return Rates

			No. of sets returned (total of 97)			
No of sets posted	No. returned	No. not returned	No controls	Both controls	Premises control only	Other control only
215	97	118	16	62	15	4

Cases occurred in all months although more cases were seen in the summer (Figure 1).

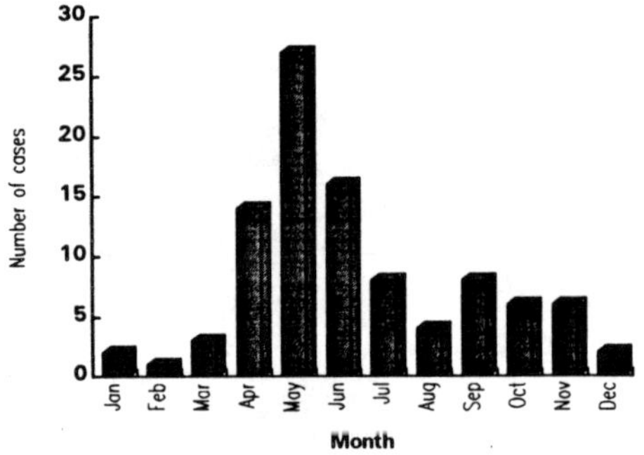

Figure 1. Occurrence of cases by month.

Univariate Statistics: The results from univariate conditional logistic regression analysis of many of the variables are recorded in Tables 3 to 5. Horse factors which appeared important at this level of analysis included the age of the horse and its condition (thin horses appeared more at risk although the numbers of thin *cases* were low). Management factors appearing important included a recent change of pasture or premises, with risk increasing as time since move decreased. The risk of grass sickness increased with increasing frequency of worming (although it was not statistically significant). Horses were at greater risk if grass sickness had previously occurred on their premises and this risk increased as the period since the last case decreased.

At this level of analysis, the sex of the horse was not associated with grass sickness, neither was its use nor was tetanus vaccination. There were no cases of grass sickness in completely stabled horses (similarly very few controls were completely stabled) and part stabling did not appear to be associated with reduced risk. Supplementary feeding similarly was not associated with a decreased risk. There was no relationship between the number of horses on the premises or in the same field and the likelihood of grass sickness. There was no association between the presence of hares or rabbits (healthy or diseased) and grass sickness. There was a tendency towards grass sickness occurring when the temperature was cool and the weather was dry although these effects were not statistically significant.

Table 3. Results from univariate analyses of horse and some management factors.

Variable	No. of Cases	Odds Ratio	p-value	95% Confidence Interval
Height (hands)	-	0.96	0.72	0.78-1.19
Age (years)	-	**0.89**	0.002	0.84-0.96
OR				
<5 years old	55	**ref**	-	-
6-10 years	25	**0.43**	0.04	0.19-0.95
>10 years	16	**0.22**	<0.001	0.09-0.50
Sex				
Gelding	50	ref	-	-
Stallion	6	1.14	0.84	0.30-4.32
Mare	35	0.79	0.48	0.41-1.52
Pregnant mare	5	1.00	1.00	0.21-4.81
OR				
Male	56	ref	-	-
Female	40	0.79	0.46	0.42-1.48
Use				
Breeding	14	ref	-	-
Pleasure Riding	41	1.31	0.66	0.40-4.37
Competing	18	0.72	0.62	0.19-2.69
Racing	4	0.83	0.84	0.15-4.63
Other	19	2.43	0.18	0.66-8.95
Worming				
{Never wormed ***	0}			
Annual worming	3	ref	-	-
6 monthly	21	0.90	0.94	0.06-13.9
2 monthly	45	2.40	0.47	0.22-26.1
more than twice monthly	25	3.41	0.32	0.30-39.1
OR				
Worming (not categorical)	-	1.69	0.10	0.91-3.16
Tetanus Vaccination	-	1.18	0.22	0.91-1.53
Condition				
Fat	19	ref	-	-
Good	69	1.48	0.36	0.64-3.42
Thin	7	5.66	0.06	0.95-33.7
OR				
Thin *v.* Fat or Good	7	4.19	0.09	0.80-21.9

*** only one control (and no cases) had *never* been wormed; thus this control's value was set to missing and the reference value was put to annual worming.

Although horses in poor condition appeared more likely to be affected with grass sickness (and this included cases diagnosed by histology as well as by clinical diagnosis alone), the majority of grass sickness cases did occur in horses in good or fat condition.

The use to which horses were put did not appear to materially affect the likelihood of grass sickness. The 'other' use group, with an odds ratio of 2.43 included several young cases of grass sickness and when age was taken into account, the size of the odds ratio was reduced.

Table 4. Results from univariate analyses of management factors.

Variable	No. of Cases	Odds Ratio	p-value	95% Confidence Interval
Management				
Entirely outdoors	59	ref	-	-
Part Stabled	38	0.92	-	-
Entirely Stabled	0	-inf	-	-
OR				
Entirely outdoors	59	ref	-	-
Stabled at all	38	0.88	0.71	0.45-1.72
Supplementary Feeding				
Hay **	55	1.26	0.54	0.61-2.61
Milled Corn**	32	1.04	0.68	0.86-1.26
Other Grain**	33	0.96	0.72	0.75-1.21
Other Food**	26	1.18	0.74	0.44-3.17
OR				
Any feed bar hay**	64	1.04	0.93	0.43-2.52
OR				
Any feed incl. hay**	76	1.16	0.75	0.46-2.94
Recent Change of Pasture				
None	29	**ref**	-	-
3-6 months	8	**3.14**	0.24	0.46-21.3
2 months	9	**5.29**	0.08	0.84-33.1
1 month	6	**3.51**	0.19	0.53-23.3
less than 1 month	13	**13.96**	0.005	2.17-89.8
Within 2 weeks	32	**22.23**	<0.001	3.99-124
OR				
Not w/i 3 months	37	**ref**	-	-
1-2 months	15	**2.40**	0.11	0.82-7.00
less than 1 month	13	**8.53**	0.004	2.00-36.3
Within 2 weeks	32	**13.13**	<0.001	3.61-47.8
Recent Change of Premises				
None w/i 4 weeks	84	**ref**	-	-
w/i 3 weeks	3	**2.00**	0.62	0.13-32.0
w/i 2 weeks	7	**4.86**	0.07	0.87-27.1
w/i 1 week	2	**4.29**	0.29	0.29-64.2
AND				
not w/i 6 months	69	**ref**	-	-
2-5 months	6	**1.11**	0.87	0.34-3.63
1 month	9	**6.54**	0.04	1.09-39.4
< 1 month	12	**5.37**	0.03	1.22-23.6

**presence versus absence of individual feed.

Recent change of both pasture and premises are associated with increased risk of grass sickness, although in multivariate analysis the effects of moving premises were reduced by adjusting for the effects of changing pasture.

Table 5. Results from univariate analyses of premises and weather factors.

Variable	No. of Cases	Odds Ratio	p-value	95% Confidence Interval
Previous g.s. on premises	41	**4.52**	0.008	1.49-13.7
premises controls excluded	41	**10.33**	0.002	2.37-45.1
Time of previous grass sickness				
no previous g.s.	55	**ref**	-	-
Yes but date unknown	3	**3.13**	0.28	0.40-24.7
>6 years ago	15	**6.49**	0.04	1.11-37.9
within 2 years	23	**9.99**	0.01	1.69-59.2
premises controls excluded				
Yes but date unknown	3	**2.41**	0.52	0.17-35.2
>6 years ago	15	**10.63**	0.03	1.22-92.4
within 2 years	23	**35.71**	0.006	2.78-458.2
In contact with previous cases of grass sickness	9	1.63	0.42	0.49-5.42
(prems with no prev gs excluded)	9	0.74	0.70	0.16-3.45
On premises at time of grass sickness	13	1.40	0.56	0.45-4.38
(prems with no prev gs excluded)	13	0.42	0.32	0.08-2.26
Grazing same field as where case occurred	13	3.01	0.07	0.92-9.84
(prems with no prev gs excluded)	13	1.34	0.76	0.21-8.47
No. horses on same premises	-	1.07	0.48	0.89-1.29
No. horses same field	-	1.09	0.35	0.90-1.32
Rabbits not seen	15	ref	-	-
seen	65	1.15	0.80	0.38-3.45
seen and sick	17	2.25	0.36	0.39-12.8
Hares not seen	60	ref	-	-
seen	33	0.90	0.80	0.40-2.03
seen and sick	3	0.18	0.13	0.02-1.65
Weather				
dry	63	ref	-	-
showery	14	0.23	0.26	0.02-2.97
wet	18	0.72	0.80	0.06-9.47
OR showery/wet (*v.* dry)	32	0.37	0.37	0.04-3.21
hot	18	ref	-	-
warm	39	0.99	0.99	0.14-6.85
cool	38	1.92	0.63	0.14-26.6
OR cool (*v.* hot/warm)	38	1.92	0.61	0.15-24.1

As controls were matched on date and many also on premises, the effects of the factors in Table 5 are expected to be artificially reduced as they assess aspects of the premises. For example, when controls from the same premises are excluded, the odds ratios associated with time of previous grass sickness and previous disease alone increase substantially.

Multivariate Analysis: A multivariate model was fitted as described and the results are presented in Table 6. Several of the factors which appeared important in the univariate analyses lost their effects after inclusion in the multivariate model. In contrast, several of the factors which appeared of no or little importance took on greater significance in the multivariate model. All variables included produced fairly stable effects which were not significantly altered by the exclusion of sets with the poorest fit (as demonstrated by the magnitude of their delta-betas).

Table 6. Results from Multivariate Analysis.

Variable	Odds Ratio	p-value	95% Confidence Interval
Time of previous grass sickness			
no previous g.s.	**ref**	-	-
Yes but date unknown	**1.70**	0.75	0.06-46.8
>6 years ago	**24.40**	0.02	1.74-341
within 2 years	**40.99**	0.005	3.11-539
Age (years)			
<5 years old	**ref**	-	-
6-10 years	**0.49**	0.20	0.17-1.47
>10 years	**0.11**	<0.001	0.03-0.39
Recent Change of Pasture			
Not w/i 3 months	**ref**	-	-
1-2 months	**8.22**	0.02	1.39-48.8
less than 1 month	**13.60**	0.03	1.24-149
Within 2 weeks	**171.1**	<0.001	14.7-1986
Worming			
(serial, not categorical)	**7.07**	0.004	1.86-26.9
Condition			
Fat or Good	**ref**	-	-
Thin	**11.3**	0.05	0.99-128
Sex			
Male	**ref**	-	-
Female	**0.28**	0.02	0.09-0.84

The effects of worming are included as a single serial variable. In fact, if worming was fitted as a categorical variable (Table 7), the effect increased with increasing frequency of worming.

Table 7. The Association between Grass Sickness and Frequency of Worming, adjusted for other variables as in Table 5.

Variable	Odds Ratio	p-value	95% Confidence Interval
Worming			
Annual worming	ref	-	-
6 monthly	6.3	0.54	0.02-2330
2 monthly	71.3	0.14	$0.23\text{-}0.22 \times 10^5$
more than twice monthly	360.9	0.05	$0.30\text{-}0.15 \times 10^6$

Power Calculations. Using the tables in Breslow and Day (1980) for sample sizes in matched case control studies, it was found that the study had a chance of more than 80% of detecting the significantly ($\alpha=0.05$) increased risks observed for all of the variables in multivariate model (Table 6).

In contrast to those factors in the multivariate model, the study was not large enough to detect any significant effects of several other variables and so their omission from the final model may have more to do with design considerations rather than absence of effect. The required number of cases is shown in Table 8.

Table 8. Sample size calculations for some effects not in final model.

Variable	Odds Ratio	p-value	No. of Cases	No. sets required to reach $\beta=0.80$, $\alpha=0.05$.
In contact with previous cases of g.s.	**0.1**	0.1	9	113
Weather cool (*v.* hot/warm)	**1.85**	0.85	38	122
Weather dry (*v.* showery/wet)	**0.09**	0.77	63	19
Height (< 15hh *v.* ≥15hh)	**1.58**	0.49	59	417
serial	**1.25**	0.24	-	
Part Stabling (*v.* Entirely Out)	**1.83**	0.41	38	122

DISCUSSION.

The quality of the completed returns was encouraging. Virtually no answers were ambiguous or inconsistent. The only real problem encountered was four owners filling in all three questionnaires for their case of grass sickness, or owners only returning a completed questionnaire from the case.

Many of the positive results are in general agreement with those previously reported by Gilmour and Jolly (1974) and Doxey *et al* (1991a). Consistent findings included an association with previous occurrence of grass sickness on the premises, which increased in strength as the period since the previous case reduced, that younger horses were at greater risk and that horses that had recently moved premises or pasture were at greater risk.

Findings that were not consistent with those of Gilmour and Jolly (1974) included that mares were at less risk than male horses. In this study, sex only became statistically significant during multivariate analysis with the univariate analysis of sex not showing a significant association. It is interesting to note that multivariate analysis of Gilmour and Jolly's data shows that mares may be at slightly reduced risk when compared to males (OR=0.66, p=0.08; S.Edwards and J.L.N.Wood, *unpublished observations*).

Gilmour and Jolly (1974) found that stabled or partly stabled horses were at reduced risk of grass sickness when compared to those at grass. In contrast, no cases of grass sickness were found in entirely stabled horses in this study and stabling was not associated with reduced risk, as also found by Doxey *et al* (1992a). Similarly, Gilmour and Jolly (1974) showed reduced risk to be associated with feeding of hay and concentrates, whereas this study shows no such difference. The reasons for these differences are not clear but include the fact that this study draws its subjects from a different geographic area where management may be different and the fact that Gilmour and Jolly's study did not collect control data at the same time as the case data.

The finding that increasing frequency of worming is associated with risk of grass sickness is novel. It would be appear to be a true effect rather than spurious for a number of reasons. Many horse owners worm their horses on moving them and as there is a very strong association between moving horses and likelihood of grass sickness, there is a possibility of some residual confounding (Davey-Smith and Phillips, 1992) However, this confounding is probably not the cause of the association, or the effects of worming would be stronger at the univariate level than in the model; moreover, the effects of worming are increased by inclusion of recent change of pasture in the model, rather than decreased as would occur with residual confounding. Additionally, there is a biological gradient with the odds ratio increasing consistently with frequency of worming.

There are two ways of interpreting this. One is that it is a direct effect, for example that the frequent removal of worms from the gut wall results in a disruption that in some way increases the absorbance of a causative agent. The other way of interpreting this is that the worming is acting as a surrogate measure for another factor. A possible example of this might be that grass sickness is associated with ingestion of a substance from the soil (rather than herbage) and that a short sward might thus predispose to the disease; owners of horses grazing such heavily cropped land might feel their horses to be at greater risk of parasitism and hence worm them more frequently. Any association between the disease and grazing density will be investigated at a later date (appropriate data for this have been recorded, although sward height itself was not recorded). It seems most unlikely that the anthelmintics themselves actually contain a substance that directly causes grass sickness, although the anthelmintic used was not recorded.

It is quite possible that factors within the intestine are important, not just due to the above finding, but also due to the fact that the figures shown by Gilmour and Jolly (1974) show an increased risk associated with the feeding of concentrate (in the absence of hay); this effect is still evident after multivariate analysis (*unpublished observations*).

Many different factors were examined in this study and so a statistically significant association between one or more variable where there is no biological association might be expected. In fact, tetanus vaccination within the previous six months appeared to be an example of this. Although significantly associated with grass sickness in multivariate analysis, the association was extremely unstable and removal of 2 matched sets with large delta-betas for this variable resulted in loss of statistical significance.

When information from further matched sets is available, other factors may become statistically significant. The calculation shown in Table 8 suggest that a further fifty matched sets may be required for the study to have adequate power to detect the effect of some of these variables.

This study has included cases of grass sickness that were diagnosed clinically by veterinary surgeons as well as those confirmed by histopathology. Future analyses will evaluate whether confirmed cases produce the same results as those diagnosed clinically. In addition, a separate analysis which only includes the controls from other premises will be carried out to better assess the size of risk associated with previous occurrence of the disease on the premises. Rather than comparing the weather conditions with those from the controls matched on date (all) and premises (half), more appropriate comparisons could be made with a national or local weather database, such as used by Doxey *et al* (1992b). The final results will be compared to those from an identical study of 'mal seco' (Uzal *et al.*, 1991; 1992) currently underway in Patagonia.

ACKNOWLEDGEMENTS

The help of owners and veterinary surgeons who participated in this study is gratefully acknowledged. John Gilmour was instrumental in helping to set this study up shortly before his death and many thanks are due to him. The study was supported by the Equine Grass Sickness Fund in particular with the help of Mr K. Scott. JLNW is supported by the veterinary advisory committee of the Horserace Betting Levy Board.

REFERENCES

Breslow, N.E. and Day, N.E. (1980). Statistical methods in cancer research. The analysis of case control studies. IARC, Lyon, 1980.

Davey-Smith, G. and Phillips, A.N. (1992). Confounding in epidemiological studies; why 'independent effects' may not be all they seem. *British Medical Journal* **305**; 757-759.

Dean, A.D., Dean, J.A., Burton, J.H. and Dicker, R.C. (1990) Epi Info, Version 5: a word processing, database and statistic program for epidemiology on microprocessors. Centers for Disease Control, Atlanta, Georgia, U.S.A.

Doxey, D.L.. Gilmour, J.S., & Milne, E.M. (1991a) A comparative study of normal equine grass sickness and those with grass sickness (dysautonomia) in eastern Scotland). *Equine veterinary Journal* **23**, 365-369.

Doxey, D.L.. Gilmour, J.S., & Milne, E.M. (1991b) The relationship between meteorological features and equine grass sickness (dysautonomia). *Equine veterinary Journal* **23**, 370-373.

Doxey, D.L., Pogson, D.M., Milne, E.M., Gilmour, J.S. and Chisholm, H.K. (1992) Clinical equine dysautonomia and autonomic neuron damage. *Research in Veterinary Science* **53**, 106-109.

EGRET (1989) Statistics and Epidemiology Research Corporation, Seattle, Washington, USA.

Gilmour, J.S. & Jolly, G.M. (1974) Some aspects of the epidemiology of equine grass sickness *Veterinary Record* **95**, 77-80.

Gilmour, J.G. (1975a) Chromatolysis and axonal dystrophy in the autonomic nervous system in grass sickness of equidae. *Neuropathology and Applied Neurobiology* **1**, 39-47.

Gilmour, J.G. (1975b) Studies in Equine Grass Sickness. Fellowship Thesis, Royal College of Veterinary Surgeons.

Greig, J.R. (1942) Grass sickness in horses. *Transactions of Royal Highland Agricultural Society* **46**, 1-27.

Obel, A.L. (1955) Studies on grass disease: the morphological picture with special reference to the vegetative nervous system. Journal of Comparative Pathology 65, 336-346.

Pool, W.A. (1927) Grass disease of horses. Paper presented to the Scottish branch of the National Veterinary Medical Association. Published as a pamphlet by A.D.R.A., Edinburgh.

Uzal, F.A., Robles, C.A. & Olaechea, F.V. (1991) Primera descripcion de alteraciones histopatologicas en los ganglios celiaco-mesenterico anteriores de un equino con 'mal seco'. *Revista de Medecina Veterinaria* **72**, 68-69.

Uzal, F.A., Robles, C.A. & Olaechea, F.V. (1992) Histopathological changes in the coeliaco-mesenteric ganglia of horses with 'mal seco', a grass sickness like syndrome, in Argentina. *Veterinary Record* **130**, 244-246.

MODELLING THE EQUINE SARCOID

REID, S.W.J.* AND GETTINBY, G.**

The equine sarcoid is an infiltrative fibropapilloma putatively caused by a papillomavirus that affects the skin of horses, donkeys and mules (Jackson, 1936; Ragland et al., 1970; Howarth, 1990; Reid, 1992). Although the tumour has a high incidence rate relative to other neoplastic diseases, epidemiological investigations have been hindered by the low prevalence of the tumour and the difficulty in obtaining population data. Previous studies have reported on the epidemiology of the sarcoid exclusively in populations of horses (Ragland et al., 1966; James, 1968; Lazary et al., 1985; Angelos et al., 1988). We have recently reported on the epidemiology of the disease in a single population of donkeys (Reid et al., 1994). This paper describes one approach to modelling the sarcoid using the same population data. A log linear model is used to describe the interaction of certain explanatory variables in the donkeys with sarcoids, that is the diseased population.

MATERIALS AND METHODS

Definition of study population

The study was based on the clinical observations in a large population of donkeys kept at The Donkey Sanctuary, Sidmouth, Devon. The definition of the study population has been described previously (Reid et al., 1994). Briefly, animals that developed sarcoid tumours were identified by screening the computerised health records of The Donkey Sanctuary from the period 1967-1990. As fibropapillomas may take up to six months to develop following inoculation (Voss, 1969), animals that had been at the Donkey Sanctuary for less than six months were excluded from the study unless they were born there. Animals that had spent time away from the Sanctuary following admission but which had subsequently returned were also excluded as these animals may have developed sarcoids due to factors or agents encountered outwith the Sanctuary.

Modelling protocol

The variables used in the present study were gender, age at first exposure (i.e., age at entry to the Sanctuary) and duration of exposure (i.e., time spent at the Sanctuary), all of which were independent. The age at which animals developed a sarcoid was not used in the modelling process as this variable was directly related to age at first exposure and duration of exposure, i.e., old animals entering the Sanctuary will be older animals when they exhibit clinical signs of the disease; older animals may have been exposed for longer. Classification tables containing counts of

*Veterinary Informatics and Health Group, Department of Veterinary Medicine, University of Glasgow Veterinary School, Bearsden Road, Bearsden, Glasgow, G61 1QH.
**Veterinary Informatics and Health Group, Department of Statistics and Modelling Science, University of Strathclyde, Glasgow, G1 1XH.

the number of diseased animals were generated for each possible combination of the levels of gender, age at first exposure and duration of exposure. The tables were condensed when the data were too sparse to allow analysis. The distribution of the number of cases amongst animals with sarcoids obtained in the multidimensional contingency table were explored using a log-linear regression model of the form

$$\log(n) = \text{constant} + \text{gender effect} + \text{age at first exposure effect} + \text{duration of exposure effect} + \text{interaction effects} + \text{error}$$

where n was the number of cases.

A parsimonious model consisting of those effects which best explained the number of cases was identified using backward stepwise variable selection and inspection of the scaled deviance and its associated degrees of freedom. The goodness-of-fit of the selected model was assessed by comparison of the numbers of observed and expected cases using chi-square analysis. Distributional assumptions were also tested using analysis of the differences between observed and expected data.

RESULTS

Eighty cases of sarcoid were identified in the population of 4126 donkeys on the Sanctuary records. The summary multidimensional contingency table is displayed in Table 1. Inspection of these data indicated that there were a large number of cases occurring in young male donkeys during the early years at the Sanctuary, an observation illustrated by the scatterplot of age at first exposure versus duration of exposure shown in Fig. 1.

Table 1. Distribution of male and female donkeys developing a sarcoid at The Donkey Sanctuary (i.e., Cases). The animals are classified according to the year of life during which they entered The Sanctuary and the time in years after entry during which the lesion was first observed. The square brackets contain the levels of each variable within the model.

	Age at first exposure (Years)	Duration of exposure (Years)					
		0.5 to <3 [1]		3 to <6 [2]		6 and over [3]	
		male	female	male	female	male	female
[1]	0.5 to <3	16	4	7	4	0	4
[2]	3 to <6	6	3	1	3	1	0
[3]	6 to <9	3	2	3	1	0	1
[4]	9 and over	5	4	4	3	1	4

Applying the log-linear model with a Poisson distribution and log link function, the coefficients displayed in Table 2 were generated. The maximal model, consisting of the main effects and all two-factor interactions, had a scaled deviance of 8.94 with 6 degrees of freedom which, as the scaled deviance is assumed to be distributed as X^2, did not differ significantly from the saturated model fitting the data exactly. Only the removal of the [gender x age at first exposure] interaction and the [age at first exposure x duration of exposure] interaction produced a model with no significant difference to the maximal or saturated models. The linear predictor of the parsimonious model describing the diseased animals at the Sanctuary was selected to be:

1 + gender + age at first exposure + duration of exposure + [gender x duration of exposure]

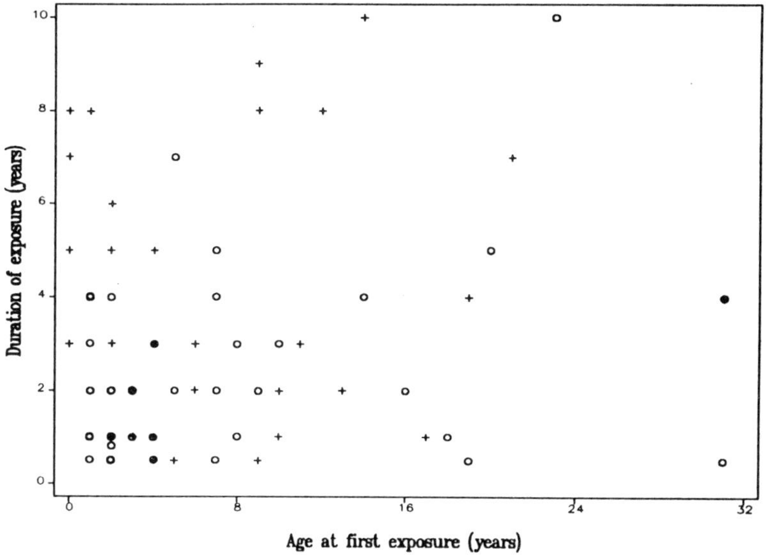

Fig 1. Scatter plot of age at first exposure versus age at entry for male (o) and female (+) donkeys with sarcoids

The coefficient and standard errors for this model are displayed in Table 2. From the table it can be seen that each of the main effects coefficients are negative values. Consequently, the prevalence of disease diminishes with being female, increasing age at first exposure and duration of exposure. In particular, males entering the Sanctuary in the first three years of life and with between 0.5 to 3 years duration of exposure appear to be at highest risk. In contrast, very few males entering between 6 and 9 years of age and with 6 to 9 years of exposure develop the disease.

However, although the risk of animals with more than 6 years of exposure is considerably diminished (coefficient -2.70), this advantage is offset in female donkeys by a large positive interaction coefficient of 2.34. Consequently, the disease is more prevalent in female donkeys with more than 6 years of exposure than in their male counterparts.

Table 2. Coefficients and standard errors for the log-linear model based on groups of animals.

Variable (level)	Coefficient	Standard error
1	2.58	0.22
gender (2)	-0.84	0.33
duration of exposure(2)	-0.69	0.32
duration of exposure(3)	-2.70	0.73
age at first exposure (2)	-0.92	0.32
age at first exposure (3)	-1.25	0.36
age at first exposure (4)	-0.51	0.28
gender(2) x duration (2)	0.53	0.52
gender(2) x duration(3)	2.34	0.85

Table 3 contains the observed and fitted counts generated by the model as well as the residuals. Figure 2 demonstrates a rankit plot of the standardised residuals confirming that they were normally distributed. Assessment of goodness-of-fit carried out by chi-square analysis indicated a good fit of the expected to observed values ($X^2 = 10.93$ with 21df).

Table 3. Observed counts, expected counts and residuals at all levels on the multidimensional contingency table, as generated by the log-linear model

Level	Males			Females		
(1st exp,dur)	Observed	Expected	Standardised residual	Observed	Expected	Standardised residual
1,1	16	13.12	0.79	4	5.69	-0.71
1,2	7	6.56	0.17	4	4.81	-0.37
1,3	0	0.88	-0.94	4	3.94	0.03
2,1	6	5.25	0.33	3	2.23	0.48
2,2	1	2.63	-1.00	3	1.93	0.78
2,3	1	0.35	1.10	0	1.58	-1.23
3,1	3	3.75	-0.39	2	1.63	0.29
3,2	3	1.88	0.82	1	1.38	-0.32
3,3	0	0.25	-0.5	1	1.13	-0.12
4,1	5	7.88	-1.03	4	3.41	0.32
4,2	4	3.94	0.03	3	2.89	0.07
4,3	1	0.53	0.66	4	2.36	1.07

DISCUSSION

This paper has described the relationship between variables significantly associated with the development of sarcoids in a diseased population. Although the model does not contain any data from control or healthy animals, the selection of the variables for inclusion in the model at the outset was based on chi-square analyses comparing sarcoid affected and unaffected donkeys. Whilst it is not possible from the analyses presented above to comment on the way the variables selected may be related to each other in the healthy population the model is a first step in a multivariate approach to an understanding of the biology of the disease.

When considering interaction terms it is important that such terms should be biologically plausible. In the present study there were a limited number of main effects and subsequently a moderate number of interaction terms to be considered. The only significant interaction term identified by the model building process was that of gender and exposure. In this case there is an effect that is greater than the additive effect of the two variables and, at first inspection, would seem to point to a significant event, occurrence or set of circumstances affecting males in particular some time after entry. Castration may be one explanation as it exclusively affects males

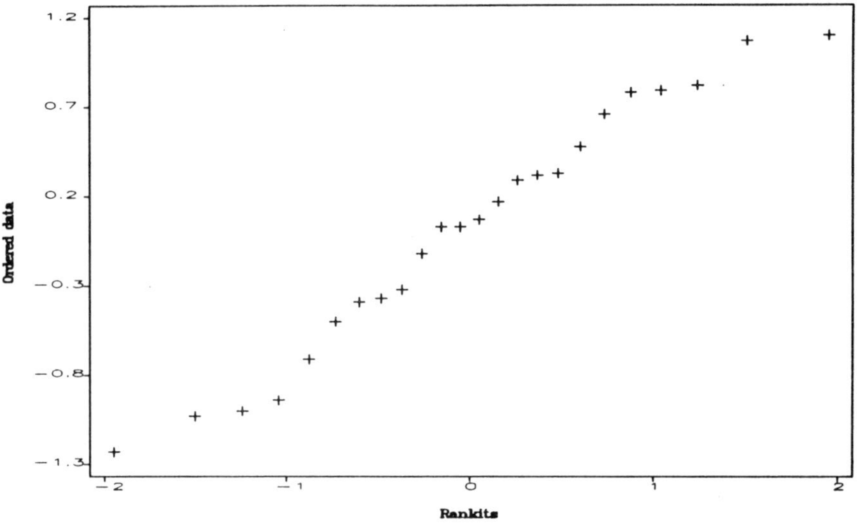

Fig.2 Rankit plot of the standardised residuals

and occurs withinthe first few months of entry to the Sanctuary. However, on inspection of the model coefficients, it is evident that the increase in occurrence of sarcoids amongst animals that develop the disease with respect to the interaction term is not associated with males but rather with females who have been at the Sanctuary for longer. This may arise because all susceptible males develop the disease earlier in life, due to unknown factors, whilst the age specific prevalence in females remains more constant throughout life. In either case, this interaction is biologically plausible and so it has remained in the model. In consideration of the other possible interactions that were not statistically significant, [age at first exposure x duration of exposure] is biologically acceptable, as this interaction may suggest an absolute age effect. However, [gender x age at first exposure] is more difficult to justify clinically and so even if this interaction had been statistically significant, there could still be grounds for excluding the term.

Even though the model has been developed on a diseased population alone, the fact that the variables involved were identified by considering both diseased and healthy donkeys means that the inferences derived may be used as a management tool. Animals that develop the disease are most likely to be young males in their first few years at the Sanctuary, an observation from the model that is in accordance with the clinical opinion. However, the model cannot be used to predict the numbers of animals in a particular population that can be expected to develop sarcoids. In order to do this, the total number of animals at risk for each combination of the explanatory variables must be included. Work is currently underway to investigate a range of models including, log-linear with Poisson distribution and including an offset value; logistic with binomial distribution using either proportions of affected animals within a group or the individual animal as the experimental unit; logistic case control based on samples of the individual animals.

The aims of any statistical model must be to increase the detection rate of disease, to diagnose disease earlier or provide an insight into the biology of the disease in the way variables interact. The model described here is a first exploratory step in this direction.

REFERENCES

Angelos, J.A., Oppenheim, Y., Rebhun, W., Mohammed, H. and Antczak, D.F. (1988) Evaluation of breed as a risk factor for sarcoid and uveitis in horses. Animal Genetics, 19, 417-425.

Howarth, S. (1990) Sarcoids: The story so far. In: The Veterinary Annual, 30th issue Eds. C.S.G. Grunsell, C.S.G. and M.E. Raw. Butterworth and Co. Ltd., London. pp145-154.

Jackson, C. (1936) The incidence and pathology of tumours of domesticated animals in South Africa. Onderstepoort J. Vet. Sci. Anim. Ind., 6, 248.

James, V.S. (1968) A familial tendency to equine sarcoids. Southwest Veterinarian, 21, 235-236.

Lazary, S., Gerber, H., Glatt, G. and Straub, R. (1985) Equine leucocyte antigens in sarcoid affected horses. Equine vet. J., 17, 283-286.

Mohammed, H.O., Rebuhn, W.C. and Antczak, D.F. (1992) Factors associated with the risk of developing sarcoid tumours in horses. Equine vet. J. 24, 165-168.

Ragland, W.L., Keown, G.H. and Gorham, J.R. (1966) An epizootic of equine sarcoid. Nature, 210, 1399.

Ragland, W.L., Keown, G.H. and Spencer, G.R. (1970) Equine sarcoid. Equine vet. J., 2, 2-11.

Reid, S.W.J. (1992) The equine sarcoid : Molecular and epidemiological studies in Equus asinus. PhD thesis, University of Glasgow.

Reid, S.W.J., Gettinby, G., Fowler, J.N. and Ikin, P. (1994) Epidemiological observations on the equine sarcoid in a population of Equus asinus. Vet. rec. (In press).

Voss, J.L. (1969) Transmission of equine sarcoid. Am. J. Vet. Res., 30, 183-191.

EPIDEMIOLOGICAL ASPECTS OF THE CONFIDENTIAL ENQUIRY OF PERIOPERATIVE EQUINE FATALITIES (CEPEF) AND SOME PRELIMINARY RESULTS

G M Johnston*

SUMMARY

The Confidential Enquiry into Perioperative Equine Fatalities (CEPEF) is an observational multi-institutional longitudinal study of recovery outcome at seven days post-operatively. An overall death rate of 151/8109 or 1.86% was established for all general anaesthetics. This mortality rate decreased to 66/7050 or 0.94% when all colic surgery was excluded.

INTRODUCTION

The sporadic nature and multifactorial aetiology of perioperative fatalities makes it impossible to design appropriate ethical or productive experimental studies, especially if no significant risk factors have been previously identified. In contrast, an epidemiological observational study of clinical cases is a more appropriate and practical investigative tool. Both anaesthetists and surgeons were involved in the present study. Steffey (1991) called for a well designed large observational study of equine anaesthesia-related morbidity and mortality.

Observational epidemiology has been used to perform comparative studies into perioperative fatalities in other species. The most closely related studies have been The Confidential Enquiries into Perioperative Deaths (Lunn & Mushin 1982, Buck et al. 1987, Campling et al. 1989, Campling et al. 1990 and Campling et al. 1993) in human surgery. Lunn and Mushin (1982) reported that one in 10,000 general anaesthetics resulted in the patient dying, purely as a result of the anaesthetic. An overall death rate of 0.7% within 30 days of surgery was identified by Buck et al. (1987), but most of the non-surviving patients were either elderly (over 75 years) or death was unavoidable due to the presenting condition, such as advanced cancer, or co-existing diseases such as cardiopulmonary failure. However the proportion of *equidae* which die unexpectedly (1.86%) is alarmingly high when it is considered that the majority of equine cases that undergo general anaesthesia for surgery are otherwise healthy and considered good surgical risks prior to surgery.

Clarke and Hall (1990) carried out a prospective survey of anaesthetic incidents and emergencies at 53 small animal practices comprising 41,881 general anaesthetics in which they found 0.15% healthy dogs and cats died primarily as a result of anaesthesia. Surgical factors were not considered.

The Animal Health Trust, PO Box 5, Newmarket, Suffolk, CB8 7DW
*

There are few reports of perioperative equine mortality surveys. Lumb and Jones (1973) published a mortality rate of 5.8% within eight days over a two year period. Tevick (1983) reported the mortality rate of 2.7% at one clinic, but these included some standing surgery. Young and Taylor (1990 and 1993) have also reported single clinic audits of equine surgery and a morbidity rate of 1.8% and a mortality rate of 0.68% respectively. The previous preliminary results from this study (Johnston 1992) showed a mortality rate of 1.79% from 62 equine clinics.

Richey et al. (1990) investigated the softer end-point of morbidity and reported the incidence of lameness after general anaesthesia to be 47/733 or 6.4% from retrospective data in one clinic. One would expect an increased morbidity rate compared to the 1.86% mortality rate reported in this paper.

Perioperative problems in all species can be subdivided into mortality and morbidity (where the patient suffers a non-life threatening complication). The central issue of a study into the incidence of perioperative problems is morbidity, but the decision as to what is included in a definition of morbidity is subjective and open to dispute. This lack of a definitive endpoint makes it difficult to collect reliable data. In contrast death provides an indisputable clearly defined endpoint as to what to include as a case in this study.

Reporting rate

In return for providing information from their clinics, all participants were thanked and sent the interim results highlighting risk factors to help reduce their incidence of perioperative fatalities. Participation in the study is voluntary. Not reporting a death would be self-defeating. A reporting rate of death of 100% was thus assumed. It is anyway more likely for a surviving case to go unreported than a non-survivor, which would only serve to strengthen further any associations shown by this study. So even if reporting rate of survivors is not complete, its effects can be ignored.

MATERIALS AND METHODS

The study population

A wide range of equine clinics and mixed practices participated. These clinics submitted information about the variety of all surgery carried out. All equine patients requiring surgery under general anaesthesia during the study period were entered into the study. The group was thus was thus exposed to a wide range of different factors with normal variation, as a result of the many different anaesthetic and surgical practices. Only cases with complete records were included in the study.

Baseline information

Each clinic was sent a package of colour coded forms relating to different aspects of equine surgery carried out at the clinic to provide information on clinic facilities; details and experience of each anaesthetist and surgeon; a brief diary for all operations under general anaesthesia and a detailed questionnaire for any perioperative fatality. This paper relates to information supplied on the diary forms only.

Confounding

The element of confounding is unknown at present. The high rate of attrition of surgical colic cases is well known to clinicians, but the influence of these cases on the overall results may become clearer in the future when the total number of general anaesthetics is sufficiently large to allow stratification of colic and non-colic surgery. Other confounding variables are unknown, but the reporting of a wide selection of potential risk factors is designed to minimise their effect.

The need to exclude pre-existing disease as a potential confounder is appreciated eg the degree of compromise experienced by many surgical colics. This has been attempted by stratification of the data on colic patients. Some tables have been compiled to show products of the stratification and indeed confirm that colic surgical patients do appear to be confounding the data and so their separate analysis is appropriate.

Error

Most of the variables were measured in a standard way by most clinicians. The forms supplied have templates and codings for all variables to maximise consistency between clinics and reduce measurement error in the method of recording variables. Such error is likely to be random rather than systematic and so maximising the number of general anaesthetics reported (i.e. increase the power of the study) is intended to reduce the effect of this error.

Follow-up

A follow-up period of seven days, was chosen because the outcome of the case would then be accurately known. This not only makes the study feasible but also maximises reporting of non-survivors. A longer period might introduce a degree of uncertainty as to a non-survivor's relationship to surgery and anaesthesia, and a shorter one might not include some of the more protracted fatal post-operative complications.

Bias

It would have been ideal, but impractical, to include all equine clinics in the country. Instead 80 clinics that carried out equine surgery were invited to participate in this voluntary survey. The validity of this type of survey depends heavily on the honesty and diligence of participating clinics. However this allows the potential for some systematic bias in that the volunteered clinics may not represent the general population of clinics carrying out equine surgery. As such the volunteer clinics can be seen as sentinel practices but any bias is assumed to be the same for survivor and non-survivors. To reduce the effect of this potential bias still further, as many of different types of equine facilities in the UK were recruited as possible.

Analysis

All data were entered onto a relational database (4th Dimension - ACIUS Inc) and were subjected to risk ratio analysis using EPI-INFO software (USD Inc, Ga USA). Each column of the diary form was analysed separately to show the numbers of surviving and non-surviving cases that were exposed to an individual risk characteristic to determine the effect of each characteristic for survivors and non-survivors.

RESULTS

These results relate to surgical procedures carried out at 62 clinics between February 1991 and September 1993.

The majority of cases (74.6%) were discharged from the clinic within seven days of surgery (table 1). A further 18.6% were still at the practice premises at seven days. 4.9% were euthanased because of inoperable lesions and 0.05% were euthanased at a subsequent surgery. The overall mortality rate was 1.86%. When all cases undergoing surgery for colic were excluded the overall mortality fell to 0.93% (50/5399).

Table 1: Overall results, outcome at seven days after surgery

	Number	%
Home	6049	74.6%
Practice Premises	1507	18.6%
Euthanasia	396	4.9%
Died	151	1.86%
Euthanasia at a later op	4	0.05%

Sex

Colts, geldings, and non pregnant females were all at similar risk (table 2). There was a twofold increase in tendency (RR=2.34) for pregnant females to die than other sex categories.

Table 2: Risk ratios for all sexes for all operations

	Total	Died	Alive	RR	95% Confid	p value
Gelding	3016	52	2964	ref		
Female	2560	58	2502	1.31	0.91-1.90	0.147
Entire male	2430	37	2393	0.88	0.58-1.34	0.56
Pregnant Subtotal	99	4	95	2.34	0.86-6.35	0.1005
Non preg sub	2461	54	2407	1.27	0.87-1.86	1.209

Table 3 shows that there was no difference in risk between non pregnant and pregnant females in their first trimester but the risk of death increased for mares throughout pregnancy. The near six fold additional risk (RR=5.47) of late term mares reached statistical significance (p=0.018).

Table 3: Risk ratios for all females for all operations

	Total	Died	Alive	RR	95% Confid	p value
1st Trimester pregnancy	57	0	57	0		
2nd Trimester pregnancy	17	1	16	2.68	0.39-18.28	0.318
3rd Trimester pregnancy	25	3	22	5.47	1.83-16.33	0.018
Non pregnant females	2461	54	2407	ref		

If colic patients were removed from the data, pregnant females had a significantly increased risk (RR=7.94, p=0.0026)

Pregnant mares were the most likely to die than any other sex category and this risk worsens as pregnancy progresses

Operation type

Colic surgery was associated with a tenfold extra risk of death (RR=10.68, p<0.0001) than the ENT group. In comparison most other surgery was associated with similar risk (table 4).

Table 4: Risk ratios for all types of surgery

	Total	Died	Alive	RR	95% Confid	p value
Orthopaedic	2822	32	2674	1.57	0.80-3.11	0.188
Colic	1059	85	974	10.68	5.73-19.90	<0.0001
Miscellaneous	881	3	878	0.45	0.13-1.62	0.21
ENT	1463	11	1452	ref		
Urogenital	1883	20	1863	1.41	0.68-2.94	0.353

Most surgery is associated with similar risk. Colic surgery is associated with significantly increased risk, much more than one would expect, when it is recalled that not all colic surgery is on moribund disasters.

Breed

Table 5 shows that the Cob would appear to be associated with extra risk. The "others" category included a number of uncommon breed types which have been grouped together.

Table 5: Risk ratios for breeds for all operations

	Total	Died	Alive	RR	95% Confid	p value
Thoroughbred	3328	56	3272	ref		
Pony	1597	31	1566	1.15	0.75-1.78	0.519
Thoroughbred Cross	1427	24	1403	1	0.62-1.61	0.99
Warm Blood	651	10	641	0.91	0.47-1.78	0.788
Hunter	287	5	282	1.04	0.42-2.56	0.813
Cob	231	10	221	2.57	1.33-4.98	0.0091
Arab	170	2	168	0.7	0.17-2.84	1
Others	413	13	400	1.87	1.03-3.39	0.037

However if colic cases were excluded, then the relative risk of Cobs return to 1.1 (table 6).

Table 6: Risk ratios for breed for non colic cases

	Total	Died	Alive	RR	95% Confid	p value
Thoroughbred	3010	30	2980	ref		
Pony	1363	10	1353	0.74	0.36-1.50	0.397
Thoroughbred Cross	1231	11	1220	0.9	0.45-1.78	0.755
Warm Blood	533	4	529	0.75	0.27-2.13	0.59
Hunter	237	1	236	0.42	0.06-3.09	0.724
Cob	183	2	181	1.1	0.26-4.55	0.705
Arab	147	2	145	1.37	0.33-5.66	0.659
Others	361	6	355	1.67	0.70-3.98	0.27

There was no obvious breed at increased risk of mortality.

Premedication

The cardiovascular compromise of many colic patients often demands a different drug regime than other types of surgery and so data from colic surgery is not presented to avoid the effect of confounding by colic patients.

Xylazine was associated with increased risk (RR=1.38) when compared to detomidine (table 7). The use of ACP, either on its own (RR=0.49, p=0.092) or in combination. was associated with decreased risk (RR=0.24, p=0.22 with xylazine or RR=0.76, p=0.45 with detomidine). Romifidine was associated with a similar reduction in risk (RR=0.5, p=0.203) as those involving ACP.

Table 7: Risk ratios for premedication for non colic patients

	Total	Died	Alive	RR	95% Confid	p value
Detomidine	1377	16	1361	ref		
ACP	1401	8	1393	0.49	0.21-1.14	0.092
ACP/Detomidine	1481	13	1468	0.76	0.36-1.56	0.45
ACP/Xylazine	357	1	356	0.24	0.03-1.81	0.22
Romifidine	689	4	685	0.5	0.17-1.49	0.203
Xylazine	873	14	859	1.38	0.68-2.81	0.37
None	84	1	83	1.02	0.14-7.63	1
Others	790	9	781	0.98	0.44-2.21	0.96

The use of ACP in non colic patients is seen to be consistently protective. The introduction of a new drug romifidine was associated with decreased risk.

Induction agents

For the same reasons as premedication, only inductions of non colic patients are shown (table 8).

80% of all inductions in non colics operations were carried out using ketamine, thiopentone, or the combination of guaiphenesin and thiopentone, and all these combinations were associated with the same or lower degree of risk (GG=Thio, RR=1.0).

In foals, inhalational halothane inductions were associated with decreased risk (RR=2.75), but there were no fatalities in this other method of inducing anaesthesia in foals.

Guaiphenesin and ketamine combination inductions were associated with increased risk (RR=4.1, p=0.04).

Table 8: Relative risk for induction agents for non colic patients

	Total	Died	Alive	RR	95% Confid	p value
Ketamine	2644	30	2614	ref		
Guaiphenesin+Thio	2228	16	2212	0.63	0.35-1.16	0.134
Thiopentone	1368	16	1352	1.03	0.56-1.88	0.92
Methohexitone	310	0	310	0		1
Valium/Ketamine	231	0	231	0		1
Inhalation Halothane	64	2	62	2.75	0.67-11.28	0.17
Guaiphenesin+Ketamine	43	2	41	4.1	1.01-16.61	0.04
Others	163	0	163	0		1

Month of surgery

The month when surgery was carried out has been grouped into quarters. Table 9 shows that a smaller proportion of operations carried out in the last quarter of the year resulted in the patient's death than in all the other quarters. This was statistically significant for each of the other quarters (p= a maximum of 0.094 for all three quarters).

Table 9: Risk ratios for season of surgery for all operations

	Total	Died	Alive	RR	95% Confid	p value
First Quarter	1563	33	1530	1.7	1.03-2.82	0.036
Second Quarter	2342	53	2289	1.83	1.15-2.89	0.009
Third Quarter	2025	38	1987	1.51	0.93-2.47	0.094
Last Quarter	2179	27	2152	ref		

It is not clear why the last quarter should be associated with a significantly decreased risk. This pattern was consistent whether colic patients were included or not.

Age of patient

Young foals carried the worst risk (RR= 8.16) and this was highly significant (p=0.0001) as shown in table 10.

Patients greater than 10 years old were associated with a relative risk of death of 3.67 and this was also significant (p=0.0005).

Table 10: Risk ratios for age of patient in all operations

	Total	Died	Alive	RR	95% Confid	p value
<1 month	103	8	95	8.16	3.02-22.02	0.0001
<6 months	438	7	431	1.68	0.59-4.75	0.324
<1 year	323	5	318	1.63	0.52-5.08	0.528
<2 years	824	8	816	1.02	0.37-2.8	0.9702
<3 years	1014	15	999	1.55	0.64-3.79	0.3291
<4 years	735	7	728	ref		
<10 years	3021	49	2972	1.7	0.77-3.74	0.179
>10 years	1315	46	1269	3.67	1.67-8.09	0.0005

The extra risks of the very young and geriatric are not surprising, and are compatible with previous reports in comparative studies in man (Lunn & Mushin 1982)

Length of anaesthesia

For non colics (table 11), after the first 30 minutes there is a tendency for risk to increase with duration of anaesthesia with the lowest risk is between 31-60 minutes (RR=0.59) and the greatest risk is between 181-240 minutes (RR=5.88, p=0.0015).

Table 11: Risk ratios for duration of anaesthesia in non colics

	Total	Died	Alive	RR	95% Confid	p value
<30 mins	1276	14	1262	ref		
31-60 mins	2024	13	2011	0.59	0.28-1.24	0.158
61-90 mins	2038	9	2029	0.4	0.17-0.93	0.39
61-120 mins	1004	12	992	1.09	0.51-2.34	0.827
121-180 mins	603	12	591	1.81	0.84-3.9	0.122
181-240 mins	93	6	87	5.88	2.31-14.95	0.0015
>241 mins	14	0	14			

The only operations lasting more than 241 minutes which died, were colics.

Start time of anaesthesia

Most surgery was carried out during normal working hours (table 12). However, the risk of dying significantly increased out of hours, especially from midnight to 7.00 am (RR=8.86, p<0.0001). Surgery carried out in the time between 17.00 and midnight also carried a relative risk of 5.65 (p<0.0001) .

Table 12: Risk ratios for starting time of anaesthesia in all operations

	Total	Died	Alive	RR	95% Confid	p value
00.01-07.00	148	14	134	8.86	5.02-15.63	<0.0001
7.01-12.00	4775	51	4724	ref		
12.01-17.00	2602	49	2553	1.77	1.19-2.60	0.0036
17.01-20.00	232	14	218	5.65	3.17-10.06	<0.0001
20.01-00.00	316	21	295	6.22	3.79-10.21	<0.0001

The relative risks remain similar when colic surgery was excluded. It may be that the particular state of many presenting colic patients may be more significant than any time factor, or perhaps these high risk patients are anaesthetised evenly throughout the twenty four hour day, and thus do not show any difference for any particular time period.

CONCLUSION

In conclusion this paper outlines the design of this multi-centred prospective observational study and provides some preliminary results which indicate the overall incidence of perioperative fatalities within seven days of surgery and highlights some relevant risk factors.

ACKNOWLEDGEMENTS

The project would have been impossible without the open mindedness, hard-work, honesty and diligence of the 62 participating practices who agreed to submit all details about their surgical practice.

This project was supported primarily by a grant from the Home of Rest for Horses with a contribution from the Association of Veterinary Anaesthetists.

Thanks are due to the Scientific Committee of The British Equine Veterinary Association and the Association of Veterinary Anaesthetists for their endorsement. The tireless good offices of Anne Campling processed and anonymised all the forms before they reached Newmarket.

Rossdale and Partners provided much encouragement and support. Computer database programming was provided by Dr Mark Holmes. James Wood provided assistance with epidemiological analysis. Dr Polly Taylor provided essential help and advice as supervisor for the project.

REFERENCES

Buck N, Devlin HB, Lunn JN (1987) The Report of a Confidential Enquiry into Perioperative Deaths. Published by the Nuffield Provincial Hospitals Trust and the King's Fund.

Campling EA, Devlin HB, Lunn JN (1989) The Report of the National Confidential Enquiry into Perioperative Deaths. Published by the Nuffield Provincial Hospitals Trust and the King's Fund.

Campling EA, Devlin HB, Hoile RW, Lunn JN (1990) The Report of the National Confidential Enquiry into Perioperative Deaths.

Campling EA, Devlin HB, Hoile RW, Lunn JN (1993) The Report of the National Confidential

Johnston GM (1991) Confidential Enquiry into Perioperative Equine Fatalities. Equine Vet Education 3, (1) 5-6

Johnston GM (1992) Proceedings of The Association of Veterinary Anaesthetists/Association of Veterinary Clinical Pharmacology and Therapeutics meeting. Glasgow.

Lunn JN, Mushin WW (1982) Mortality Associated with Anaesthesia. Published by the Nuffield Provincial Hospitals Trust.

Lumb WV, Jones EW (1973) Statistics and Records. Chapter 23 in Veterinary Anaesthesia. Lea and Febiger, Philadelphia pp 631-632. Publishing personal communiactions by Heath RB (1970) and Short CE (1970).

Powell DG (1989) The Application of Epidemiology to the Investigation of Equine Disease. Equine Vet Journal 21, (4), 237-239

Richey MT, Holland MS, McGrath CJ, Dodman NH, Marshall DB, Court MH, Norman WM, Seeler DC (1990) Equine post-anaesthetic lameness. A retrospective study. Vet Surg. 19; 392-397

Robertson JT, Beard WL (1991) Preoperative Evaluation of the Horse. Equine Anesthesia - Monitoring and Emergency Therapy. 1st Edition. Ed. Muir WW & Hubbell JAE. Published by Mosby Year Book, St Louis. pp 123.

Steffey EP (1991) Equine Anaesthesiology. Equine Vet Journal , Special supplement 11, 2-3

Steffey EP, Wheat JD, Meagher DM, Norrie RD, McKee J, Brown M, Arnold J (1977) Body position and mode of ventilation influences arterial pH, oxygen and carbon dioxide tensions in halothane-anesthetised horses. Am J Vet Res. 38; 3, 379-382

Taylor PM (1992) Risk factors and problems in Equine Anaesthesia. Proceedings of Bain-Fallon lectures. p1-5

Turner A S (1978). Surgical Complications and how to minimise them: General considerations. 24th Proc Congress AAEP 203-204.

Tevick A, (1983) The Role of Anaesthesia in Surgical Mortality in Horses. Nord Vet-Med 35, 175-179

Young SS, Taylor PM, (1990) Factors leading to serious anaesthetic related problems in equine anaesthesia. Abstract JAVA vol 17, p59

Young SS, Taylor PM (1993) Factors influencing the outcome of equine anaesthesia: a review of 1,314 cases. EVJ 25, (2) 147-151

Printed at the University of Edinburgh

SOCIETY FOR VETERINARY EPIDEMIOLOGY AND PREVENTIVE MEDICINE

APPLICATION FOR MEMBERSHIP

Name ....

Address ....

....

....

....

I wish to be elected to membership of the Society for Veterinary Epidemiology and Preventive Medicine.

Signed ....

Date ....

INTEREST GROUPS

Please tick the appropriate boxes to indicate your interests:

- ☐ Computing, including data-logging
- ☐ Population and animal disease databases
- ☐ Sero-epidemiology
- ☐ Herd health and productivity schemes
- ☐ The economic effects of disease on animal production
- ☐ Disease nomenclature and epidemiological terminology
- ☐ Statistical techniques and modelling
- ☐ Analytical epidemiology (observational studies)
- ☐ Disease control strategies

please turn over

Please send this form to the Society's Secretary:

Dr K.S. Howe
Agricultural Economics Unit
Economics Department
University of Exeter
St German's Road
Exeter
EX4 6TL

The annual subscription is £10.

SOCIETY FOR VETERINARY EPIDEMIOLOGY AND PREVENTIVE MEDICINE

CONSTITUTION AND RULES

NAME

1. The society will be named the Society for Veterinary Epidemiology and Preventive Medicine.

OBJECTS

2. The objects of the Society will be to promote veterinary epidemiology and preventive medicine.

MEMBERSHIP

3. Membership will be open to persons either actively engaged or interested in veterinary epidemiology and preventive medicine.

4. Candidates for election must return a completed application form. The Secretary will then circulate the names of candidates on the agenda for the next general meeting. Election of candidates will be by a simple majority vote of members present at the general meeting.

5. Non-payment of subscription for six months will be interpreted as resignation from the Society.

OFFICERS OF THE SOCIETY

6. The Officers of the Society will be President, Senior Vice-President, Junior Vice-President, Honorary Secretary and Honorary Treasurer. Officers will be elected annually at the Annual General Meeting, with the exception of the President and Senior Vice-President who will assume office. No officer can continue in the same office for longer than six years.

COMMITTEE

7. The Executive Committee of the Society normally will comprise the officers of the Society and not more than four ordinary elected members. However, the Committee will have powers of co-option.

ELECTION

8. The election of office bearers and ordinary committee members will take place at the Annual General Meeting. Ordinary members of the Executive Committee will be elected for a period of three years. Retiring members of the Executive Committee will be eligible for re-election. Members will receive nomination forms with notification of the Annual General Meeting. Completed nomination forms, including the signatures of a proposer, seconder, and the nominee, will be returned to the Secretary at least 21 days before the date of the Annual General Meeting. Unless a nomination is unopposed, election will be by secret ballot at the Annual General Meeting. Only in the event of there being no nomination for any vacant post will the Chairman take nominations at the Annual General Meeting. Election will be by simple majority of members voting at the Annual General Meeting. Tellers will be appointed by unanimous agreement of the Annual General Meeting.

FINANCE

9. An annual subscription will be paid by each member in advance on the first day of May each year. The amount will be decided at the annual general meeting and will be decided by a simple majority vote of members present at the annual general meeting.

10. The Honorary Treasurer will receive, for the use of the Society, all monies payable to it and from such monies will pay all sums payable by the Society. He will keep account of all such receipts and payments in a manner directed by the Executive Committee. All monies received

by the Society will be paid into such a bank as may be decided by the Executive Committee of the Society and in the name of the Society. All cheques will be signed by either the Honorary Treasurer or the Honorary Secretary.

11. Two auditors will be appointed annually by members at the annual general meeting. The audited accounts and balance sheet will be circulated to members with the notice concerning the annual general meeting and will be presented to the meeting.

MEETINGS

12. Ordinary general meetings of the Society will be held at such a time as the Executive Committee may decide on the recommendation of members. The annual general meeting will be held in conjunction with an ordinary general meeting.

GUESTS

13. Members may invite non-members to ordinary general meetings.

PUBLICATION

14. The proceedings of the meetings of the Society will not be reported either in part or in whole without the written permission of the Executive Committee.

15. The Society may produce publications at the discretion of the Executive Committee.

GENERAL

16. All meetings will be convened by notice at least 21 days before the meeting.

17. The President will preside at all general and executive meetings or, in his absence, the Senior Vice-President or, in his absence, the Junior Vice-President or, in his absence, the Honorary Secretary or, in his absence, the Honorary Treasurer. Failing any of these, the members present will elect one of their number to preside as Chairman.

18. The conduct of all business transacted will be under the control of the Chairman, to whom all remarks must be addressed and whose ruling on a point of order, or on the admissibility of an explanation, will be final and will not be open to discussion at the meeting at which it is delivered. However, this rule will not preclude any member from raising any question upon the ruling of the chair by notice of motion.

19. In case of an equal division of votes, the Chairman of the meeting will have a second or casting vote.

20. All members on election will be supplied with a copy of this constitution.

21. No alteration will be made to these rules except by a two-thirds majority of those members voting at an annual general meeting of the Society, and then only if notice of intention to alter the constitution concerned will have appeared in the notice convening the meeting. A quorum will constitute twenty per cent of members.

22. Any matter not provided for in this constitution will be dealt with at the discretion of the Executive Committee.

April, 1982
Revised March, 1985; April, 1988